LIFE AFTER DEATH

By Robert C. Fischer

With special thanks to Elizabeth Ridley (editor)!

Her skills kept my writing professional.

This story is a true account of real-life occurrences as remembered by Robert and his wife, Carole.

To my loving wife, Carole, who makes all my happiness possible.

Contents

Prologue

The following is my personal account of experiencing and coping with an aortic aneurysm and dissection. It is a rare, life-threatening medical emergency, and mine came completely without warning. One of the terrifying things about it was that I was completely unaware for months or even years before that I even had an underlying condition, a condition ready to burst, ready to kill me. My emergency could have easily happened at any time, at a time that wouldn't have been so good. This is one reason why the potential consequence of this *event* is usually lethal. Plus, as will be seen with my story, the trauma from this *event* can lead to subsequent complications, compounding the damage. But one of the worst things from going through this is that it is something from which I will never be fully healed. It will be with me for the rest of my life.

That's part of the reason for choosing the title of this book, *Life After Death*. Besides the literal reason of surviving two cardiac arrests, the more meaningful reason is that my life after my *event* has changed so significantly that it is almost like losing the life I had before.

I hope by writing about my experience it will bring awareness about this emergency, and to offer others knowledge about what might be expected if they would ever encounter it. It is survivable. But it requires responsiveness, not only from the person who has the emergency, but also from the personnel at the ER in recognizing the emergency.

Also, I wish to thank my dear wife, Carole, for all of her love and support. She was pushed beyond her limits, having to deal with things she never wished to deal with in her life. She has been amazing. I could not have survived this ordeal without her. She is my true love.

Finally, one thing as you read this book. Please note that the things that happened to me are neither better nor worse than what others have experienced with this deadly *event*. It is merely my own personal story.

Which all started with an...

CHAPTER 1: Emergency

It was Tuesday, August 2, 2016. It will be a date that I'll never forget. I was fifty-five years old at the time, and I was in fair-to-good health. Or, at least like most people, I thought I was. It wasn't that I didn't have medical issues; they just weren't critical, nothing to be overly concerned about.

I had gotten up for work like most days. I made the bed, showered, ate breakfast with my loving wife, cleaned the cat's litter box, and went outside in the hot Texas summer weather to get the daily newspaper. Nothing out of the ordinary. Nothing to worry about. Everything seemed fine. Again, just another typical workday.

The time was about 7:00 a.m., and I was five minutes away from leaving the house. I was in the bathroom brushing my teeth, the last thing in my ritual of getting ready for the day. Afterward, it would just be a matter of saying goodbye to my wife, Carole, and my cat, Pippin. Then, off to work.

[I'm retired now, but back then I worked for the Boeing Company, which is about a half-hour commute from my house in League City, Texas, a suburb halfway between Houston and Galveston.]

Lucky for me, I was not yet on my way to work, driving alone in my car. If I had been, I don't think I would be here telling this story.

I had just put my toothbrush away, and that's when it happened. Without any warning or prior symptom, I was struck with a sudden, intense pain in my chest. I reeled from the shock of it. Besides a feeling of extreme tightness, as if I were having a charley horse in my chest muscles, there was also a burning, tearing sensation, like something being ripped apart inside my chest. I was in a lot of pain, and panic immediately set in. There was no mistaking that something terrible had just happened. This wasn't heartburn. This wasn't indigestion. My first thought was that I was having a heart attack. Frightened, but still able to walk, I made my way into the living room to find Carole.

I didn't want to scare Carole, but I knew I needed help – immediately! I tried to think of the least alarming way to explain to her that I thought I needed to go to the hospital, but I couldn't think of anything quickly to soften the news. So, I straightforwardly told her that I was having this terrible pain across my chest. She could tell from my expression that there was something serious going on. She asked me to describe the pain. I didn't know what to say except that my chest really hurt and that it felt wrong, that it was something I never felt before. I sat down in our armchair and held my chest.

Since there had been a time before when I had gone to the ER after experiencing a numbing, tingling pain in my left arm, but it turned out to be an anxiety attack, Carole wasn't sure what was going on. So, she asked if I thought I really needed to go to the hospital. Since I knew this was different, something bad, I reluctantly said yes. She could tell that I was scared. I also felt scared for her. I hated having her worry.

Carole then asked if I needed an ambulance or would it be okay for her to drive me to the emergency room. With the pain not getting any worse, I felt that it was okay to drive there ourselves. So, Carole told me that she needed to go and get dressed. She rushed back into our bedroom.

Feeling a bit uneasy, I lay down upon our living room floor. I was still thinking that I was having a heart attack. So did Carole, for she soon came back and handed me an aspirin to swallow. I could see the panic in her face, and I could hear it in her voice. I tried to remain calm for her, even though my own fear was escalating. As Carole left again to get dressed, she kept talking with me. I later found out that she was making sure that I was still okay. It would turn out to be a good thing she did, because I eventually passed out. I soon awoke to Carole frantically calling my name, urging me to regain consciousness, yelling for me not to die on her. She told me that I had passed out. I denied it, though I could not remember the last minute or so. Now beyond worried, she gave up the notion of driving me to the hospital and called 911.

This is where my memory of the day becomes unclear. I remember the two EMTs coming into our house, bending over me on the floor, and asking me what happened and how I felt. They were very calm and talked to me nonchalantly, trying to ease both Carole's and my fear. I told them about the pain in my chest and how I thought that the pain may have been subsiding. Thinking about it now, I'm not sure if I was really feeling better or if I was just hoping that I was, for my sake and for Carole's. I do remember thinking that Carole must have been freaking out and I had wanted her to worry less. I was feeling bad for her.

Once the situation was explained, the EMTs took my blood pressure and checked other vital signs. I heard Carole telling them that I had passed out, which I still didn't fully realize because my mind was now a bit fuzzy. I did understand that things were not good, but I felt better knowing that at least professional help was there.

But it wasn't until the EMTs said that they would be taking me to the hospital that it confirmed my situation. I couldn't believe this was happening. And with my mind a bit out of it, this felt more like a dream. Was this for real?

After getting me onto a gurney, the EMTs wheeled me out of the house and into the ambulance. I remember wondering if anyone in the neighborhood was watching. I was one of the younger members in our 55+ community, and I thought how ironic it was that I was the one being placed into an ambulance.

Never having been in an ambulance before, I was both intrigued and scared. However, as I lay there waiting to leave, I started thinking about the enormity of the situation. Realizing how serious this was, I think I started going into shock. What the hell was going on? Just how serious was this? I finally began to think, was I going to die?

The ambulance did not depart immediately. I didn't know why, but I kept wondering what's the delay. While waiting, I noticed that my right hip began to hurt. The pain wasn't too bad, at least not yet, so I didn't think much about it. After another minute or two, the ambulance finally began moving and soon I was on my way to Methodist St. John Hospital, which is probably about a twenty-minute ride away with normal traffic and lights. Once outside my neighborhood, I heard the sirens turn on. It reinforced to me how critical things were. I still couldn't believe this was real.

En route to the hospital, my chest pain gave way to an excruciating pain in my right hip and leg. The pain was not sharp, but it was strong and uncomfortable, as if someone jammed a large metal ball underneath my upper leg muscle and then pressed down hard on it. It was the type of pain that grew over time, becoming more unbearable with each passing minute. I began crying out from the pain. Strange that it didn't even occur to me to wonder what might have been causing the pain. I would find out later that the hip and leg pain was due to a lack of blood flow to my leg muscle.

~~~~~~~~~~~~~

While I was being taken to the hospital, Carole contacted her daughter, Jennifer, to let her know about what was going on. Jennifer was shocked and worried. However, she lived in Dallas and
~~~~~~~~~~~~~

was unable to be there for Carole anytime soon. So, Jennifer did the next best thing. Not telling Carole of her plans, Jennifer phoned Tobie, a friend of Carole's, and asked her if she could go to the hospital to be with Carole. Of course, Tobie said yes, and she and her husband, Jim, headed straightaway to St. John Hospital. As will be seen, I am so glad that Jennifer had the forethought to call Tobie.

As Carole was on her way to the hospital, Jennifer called her mom back, and told her that even though she may get mad about it, she had called Tobie to meet her at the hospital for support. Carole thought it was unnecessary to bother Tobie, especially since I had told her that I was feeling better. At this point, Carole wasn't positive that I was even having a heart attack. However, Carole would be very grateful later. Regardless, having Tobie and Jim with her at the hospital did provide her comfort.

[A humorous side note: With this being an emergency, neither Carole nor Tobie had time to do their usual morning preparedness. So, for all their time that they would spend at the hospital this day, neither woman sported makeup, which for them is a major ordeal. Carole to this day tells me I owe her for that.]

~~~~~~~~~~~~~

From here on, my memory is sketchy at best. It was now sometime between 8:00 and 9:00 in the morning. I don't remember getting to the hospital, or talking with any of the doctors or nurses, or even having an examination done. I do have a vague recollection of begging incessantly for pain medication for my leg and hip, as the pain had become intolerable. But apparently, the doctors could not give me pain medications yet until they figured out what was going on. This will be my last memory of the day, even though Carole later told me I was awake throughout the time until my surgery, which would be hours later.

[Another humorous side note: As I was lying on a hospital bed in one of those flimsy hospital gowns (I don't remember ever getting into the gown), I kept tossing and turning due to my leg and hip pain. Carole kept telling me to settle down,
~~~~~~~~~~~~~

that my movement would make my condition worse. Someone may have told me what my condition was, but at that point in time I had no comprehension of what was going on. As such, I was more engrossed with my pain than being compliant in lying still. What I also didn't realize was that Tobie had arrived and was by Carole's side. So, each time I tossed and turned, I ended up exposing my naked butt to the both of them. Of course, I didn't care about that either, considering my pain. This would be a good laugh later. Much later.]

What I would eventually learn about what happened to me is that the ER doctor at St. John Hospital, Dr. Denise Ryan, had the insight to suspect my condition – an aortic dissection due to aneurysm. This is a rare and usually fatal condition, one that many doctors will never encounter. Therefore, some don't consider it. Since my event, I have heard a few horror stories about how some doctors misdiagnose the symptoms of an aortic dissection. Apparently, once a heart attack is ruled out and not having any other indicative lab results, some doctors chalk up the chest pain to indigestion or some other minor condition. The patient may even be sent home, which is dire considering how time-sensitive an aortic dissection and aneurysm can be.

This time, however, I was one of the lucky ones. I am so grateful that the staff at St. John Hospital was aware of the possibility. Having checked my blood pressure, the ER nurse saw that the pressure in my one arm was significantly different than my other arm – an indicator of an aortic dissection. Without delay, Dr. Ryan ordered a CT scan to confirm.

Once my condition was confirmed by the scan, Carole was told that I needed cardiac surgery – *now!* In fact, I was to be life-flighted to Houston Methodist Hospital in the Texas Medical Center since I needed a specialist for this type of surgery. Carole was in disbelief. She and her friend Tobie just looked at one another. I had gone from a possible heart attack to a life-threatening situation where each second counted. Carole was told to leave now to get to Houston Methodist Hospital since life-flight would get me there much more quickly. It is about an hour's drive by car into Houston and only about a twenty-minute helicopter flight. Thank God that she had Jim and Tobie to drive her there. Thank God Jennifer called Tobie. I can't imagine the anxiety that Carole must have been facing right then. I often wonder how I would have reacted if the situation was reversed, and Carole was the one on the verge of dying.

~~~~~~~~~~~~

With Jim driving, Carole finally had the opportunity to call another one of her friends, Allyson, who also happened to be a nurse with considerable medical knowledge and ER experience. Unfortunately, Allyson was out of town on travel, but Allyson still was able to provide Carole some comfort over the phone, trying to explain to her what was going on. After all, how many people have ever heard of an aortic dissection? Even so, Carole only half heard what was said since everything had become a blur for her, as all kinds of scary thoughts raced through her head.

Through the following days, Carole would rely on Allyson's support. One thing Allyson warned her, though, was, "Things will get worse before they start getting better." How true those words came to be.

~~~~~~~~~~~~

After a seemingly long, anxious trip, Carole finally arrived at Houston Methodist Hospital and began searching for me. However, she was told that I was not there yet; my life-flight trip had gotten delayed. To this day, I have no clue as to what caused the delay. I can't imagine what must have been going on in Carole's mind, thinking about all the possible reasons why I hadn't arrived yet. Those mind gerbils racing on those treadmills of worry are infamous at coming up with all sorts of possibilities. I mean, who would have thought that a car would beat a helicopter?

In time, I would finally arrive. But after waiting for what must have seemed like an eternity, and with no information coming from the hospital, Carole eventually had to ask again where I was. This time, she was directed to the room where I was being prepped for surgery. Besides being able to see me, this would turn out to be a good thing since she was able to answer questions that the hospital had for me, for I was not coherent enough to be of much help.

When I was finally ready for surgery, Carole wished me well. Still out of it, either from the pain or from the dissection itself, I was not very responsive to Carole, something I regret to this day. This would be the last time Carole would see me before surgery, and she was worried beyond belief. What if this really would be the last time that she ever saw me alive? And here I was unable to comfort her or tell her how much I loved her. Unfortunately, I don't remember any of that. I wish I could. However, as I already said, I don't recall anything else beyond those few fuzzy moments back at St. John Hospital. Which isn't all bad, because I also don't remember anything about being transported by helicopter, which is a good thing due to my fear of heights.

Surgery and Cardiac Arrest #1

As it turned out, my luck would still be with me. One of the best cardiac surgeons in the world, Dr. Michael Reardon, was there to operate on me. He trained under the famous Dr. Denton Cooley, and he is an expert in aorta repair surgery.

Curious, Tobie's husband, Jim, asked Dr. Reardon just how many of these surgeries had he performed. Dr. Reardon answered hundreds, and he just did one two days prior. Being the kidder that Jim was, Jim gave Dr. Reardon his personal seal of approval, saying that he guessed it would be okay then for Dr. Reardon to perform my surgery.

[*As will be seen, Dr. Reardon was a godsend. Besides his cardiac surgery expertise, he is a very caring person, as evident in his bedside manner, especially with how he comforted Carole.*]

Before performing my surgery, Dr. Reardon explained to Carole about what my surgery would entail, even drawing a crude diagram of my aorta and the likely repair needed.

[*I still possess that drawing as a reminder. It is the basis for my book cover.*]

One of the things that he informed her about was that because of the expected trauma done by the dissection, I would need to have my aortic valve replaced. He told her there were two options when replacing an aortic valve – a mechanical valve or a biological valve. A mechanical valve lasted longer, but the patient needed to be on blood thinners for the rest of their lives. A biological valve lasted ten to fifteen years, but it did not need blood thinners. Dr. Reardon also discussed that when the time came to replace a biological valve, it would most likely be done by using a catheter going through an artery, not another invasive surgery. I learned later that this procedure is called a Transcatheter Aortic Valve Replacement (TAVR). After discussing all of this with Carole, he asked which valve did she wish to use. She had no idea which was better, so she asked Dr. Reardon what he would do. With his easy-going demeanor, Dr. Reardon said, "Well, if it was my little brother, I'd go with the biological valve." That satisfied Carole.

Before leaving, Dr. Reardon assured Carole that I would be fine, that I would survive this. I commend Dr. Reardon for being so compassionate with Carole and easing her worry. She later told me that after seeing Dr. Reardon's calm and confident attitude, she had no idea just how risky my condition really was. That's because Dr. Reardon made it sound like this was just another routine surgery for him. And, for him, it was probably true. However, I have been told since that my chance of survival that day may have been less than five percent. Not just because of the complexity of the surgery, but because many people don't even make it to surgery. I'm so glad that Carole did not know this before my surgery.

One other thing that helped keep Carole calm: While in the waiting room, the operating room liaison came and asked Carole how she was doing. The liaison also asked her who was doing my surgery. When Carole told her that it was Dr. Reardon, the liaison replied that I had one of the best surgeons. Every bit of reassurance helps.

Well, it seemed that my luck would push that low-percentage survival chance to the limit. When it came time for my surgery to begin, now about 12:00 or 12:30 p.m., I barely managed to make it into the operating room before my blood pressure crashed to zero. In other words, I had a cardiac arrest. This occurred just after being given general anesthesia. Dr. Reardon was forced to start emergency surgery, and he began cutting me open right away.

My surgery required open heart surgery, which means a sternotomy – my chest cracked open. Once my insides were exposed, Dr. Reardon discovered that the reason my heart had stopped was due to blood pooling around it. Apparently, the aneurysm at my aortic root finally ruptured, causing it to bleed, and the blood got trapped inside the sac surrounding my heart, the pericardium. The trapped blood exerted too much pressure, or tamponade, on my heart for it to be able to beat. Once Dr. Reardon cut into the pericardium to relieve the pressure, my blood pressure returned. With the immediate crisis over, Dr. Reardon could now continue on to repairing my aorta.

For the repair of my aorta, I would first need to be put on a heart/lung bypass machine. An incision was made to my front right shoulder area near the top of my pectoral muscle. A cannula, or tube, was sutured into my right subclavian artery. This tube would supply blood flow coming from the bypass machine. To return blood back to the bypass machine, a sump catheter was placed into my right superior pulmonary vein. Finally, a cardioplegic cannula was placed into my coronary sinus. This last tube would be used to supply medication directly to my heart in order to stop it. Scary thought, that my heart would purposely be stopped, and for a long period of time.

Once the bypass machine was hooked up, they began cooling my body. This was something that I never heard of before. I would find out later that a lower body temperature during cardiac surgery helps protect my heart, brain, and other organs by slowing down my metabolism and reducing the amount of oxygen needed to my organs.

The next step was to clamp off my aorta. At this point, Dr. Reardon delivered the cardioplegia medicine to my heart. He also opened up my aneurysm and checked how much damage needed to be repaired. When he did, he discovered that, besides the aortic root, the damage had extended into my left coronary artery. So, in order to repair my aorta, he would first need to cut free both of my coronary arteries, which branched off the damaged aortic root. Once severed, my left coronary artery could be repaired by placing rows of sutures in it. And, as anticipated, my aortic valve leaflets also needed to be removed for later replacement.

After about thirty minutes of cooling and after the cardioplegia medicine fully kicked in, my heart stopped. This time intentionally. Dr. Reardon could now begin repairing my aorta. Because of the aneurysm rupture, the damage was more extensive than expected. He was forced to replace the entire ascending portion of my aorta from the root to the arch. To do so, he used a Dacron graft, a synthetic material, for its replacement. I am still in awe that a tube made of synthetic material can replace someone's main blood vessel.

[An interesting side note about the Dacron graft, which I read from an article by the Houston Methodist Hospital. The Dacron graft was developed by Dr. Michael E. DeBakey at Houston Methodist Hospital. He first developed it on his wife's sewing machine. Originally, he wanted to use nylon or vinyon, the fabric used to make parachutes, but he couldn't find any at the department store. The store clerk suggested using Dacron instead. DeBakey soon realized that Dacron

was superior to nylon and vinyon since it didn't degenerate as fast over time. I think this story is amazing, considering the ingenuity of DeBakey and others like him. There is much more about doctors DeBakey and Cooley, who pioneered much of today's aortic and cardiac surgeries, but that is for others to write about.]

Once the graft was sutured in place, blood flow was resumed, and my body could start to be warmed again. Next, my new biological aortic valve was put in, but it had to be self-constructed by Dr. Reardon so it could be seated properly. Finally, my coronary arteries were reattached. Holes were cut into the Dacron graft and then the arteries were sutured on. All that was left was to wean me off the cardiopulmonary bypass machine, unhook everything, insert a chest tube, and close me up.

All in all, my surgery took about six to seven hours, and I was given many units of blood. It is unbelievable how much blood was lost and used for this surgery. But, because I was still "oozing" blood, Dr. Reardon decided not to close me up for now. Instead, he stuffed my chest cavity with surgical packing. The consequence of this was that my chest had to remain open. When I think about that now, I still find it hard to imagine being left with an open chest. It's still a bit unnerving. Anyway, Dr. Reardon planned on closing my chest the next day once he confirmed all of my bleeding had stopped. Once bandaged up (I always wondered what was used to cover my open chest), I could now be taken to the critical care ICU.

With my surgery complete, Dr. Reardon went to find Carole and tell her about my status. Besides Tobie and Jim being there with her, Carole's daughter, Jennifer, and her husband, Scott, had also now arrived from Dallas.

Dr. Reardon told Carole about the more extensive damage caused by my ruptured aneurysm, and he mentioned that my blood pressure had bottomed out. He didn't say that I had arrested, but Carole understood what he meant. He also warned her that my chest was left opened. Carole was both relieved and worried. My surgery was over, but how critical was I yet? Just what were my chances to survive? Unfortunately, this would be a lingering worry for Carole for days to come.

~~~~~~~~~~~~

Assuming that the worse was over, and with it getting late in the day, our dear friends Tobie and Jim decided to leave. They also knew that with Jennifer and Scott there, Carole would be well taken care of, including driving Carole home. I want to say just how blessed it was to have someone spend most of their day in the hospital providing support like they did. I hate to imagine if Carole had to have gone through all of this alone. And, if it wasn't for Jennifer, Carole just might have done so.

[A funny side note about our friends: Since Tobie and Jim drove Carole to Houston Methodist Hospital, Carole left her car at St. John Hospital. Because it would be very late by the time Carole returned home, Tobie and Jim told Carole not to worry about her car, that Tobie would drive her car back to our house. What they didn't realize was that Carole's car is a sports car with small seats and a small interior, which is fine for her and me, who are on the smaller size. Not quite so good for normal-sized people, especially when you can't figure out how to change the car's seat position. It must have been a humorous sight watching Tobie drive Carole's car back to our house. They are such wonderful friends.]

Cardiac Arrest #2

Not long after being put in ICU, I arrested once again. This time it would last for about fifteen minutes. Carole was taken to a room where Dr. Reardon informed her about what just happened. Again, instead of telling Carole that I had arrested, Dr. Reardon made it sound less severe by merely saying that my blood pressure went down to nothing. I thank Dr. Reardon for being so thoughtful to her. He said he needed to go back in and see what was going on. As before, Carole knew what things meant, and she was scared. I mean, who wouldn't be? To have your spouse of nearly thirty years
~~~~~~~~~~~~

seemingly barely hanging on to life, that's a lot to deal with. And, to make matters more ominous, after Dr. Reardon left, the hospital chaplain entered and asked if he could say a prayer with Carole. Carole wasn't sure what to expect now, and her fear grew, thinking that things were much more dire than she was led to believe. Learning what Carole had to go through pains me more than she'll ever know. I know how I would be if the situation was reversed.

Back in the operating room, when Dr. Reardon reopened my chest, he didn't find anything significantly wrong – no ischemia, no bleeding. He deduced that the surgical packing placed against my heart was causing tamponade, and the constriction became too great for my heart to pump, just like what happened to me when the blood from my aneurysm pooled around my heart. Once Dr. Reardon relieved the pressure, I became stable. After forty-five minutes to ensure that all was good, Dr. Reardon was satisfied that I was out of the woods. I was taken back to the ICU.

Finding Carole again, Dr. Reardon explained about the tamponade caused by the surgical packing. He also told Carole that he still intended to wait until the next morning before closing me up, but he didn't know exactly when as he had to fit me in between other scheduled patients. Again, she was relieved and grateful, but still very concerned that I was on a threshold between life and death.

After all of this drama, it was now somewhere between 10:00 p.m. and 11:00 p.m. There was nothing more that could be done besides wait and pray. Even though I survived the surgery, the hard part wasn't over, and Carole would still have to suffer through many upcoming days of agonizing worry. For today, though, it had been nearly sixteen grueling hours since this nightmare all began, and Carole was exhausted. She needed to return home for some rest. But her rest wouldn't be long, maybe for only about four hours by the time she got home and had to get back up. That's because Carole wanted to return to the hospital first thing in the morning to make sure she was there when Dr. Reardon closed me up (hopefully closed me up, if there was no further bleeding or incidents).

~~~~~~~~~~~~

Come the next morning, Carole got up early as planned and headed back to Methodist Hospital along with Jennifer and Scott. She was still worn out but managed to be there. Still scared about my delicate state of health, she couldn't wait to see me. After all, seeing is believing when your mind generates all sorts of negative thoughts.

Being in the critical care ICU, only two visitors were allowed in at a time, and only for a limited time. Carole and Jennifer were finally allowed to go in and see me. And what a sight it must have been, seeing me lying in bed, unconscious, hooked up to a multitude of equipment, along with a sign hanging over my bed stating that I had an open chest. This was tough for Carole to see. Thankfully, though, nothing of note happened to me during the brief night. I was still stable. Carole breathed a little easier.

~~~~~~~~~~~~

Once their visitation time for the morning was up, Carole and Jennifer headed back to the waiting room, somewhere they would spend a lot of time over the next few days. Carole would pass the many days ahead becoming very familiar with other parts of the hospital, including where to eat and where to pray. Many prayers were offered to God, first begging for my survival, and later hoping that I would make a full recovery.

Still early morning, Carole waited to find out about my chest closure. But as expected, it took some time before Dr. Reardon was finally able to take me back to surgery. When he did, he saw that I was doing fine. I could now be closed up. And, I must say that Dr. Reardon did a remarkable job. Much later, when I finally had a chance to look at my incision wound, I saw that my scar was hardly noticeable. In fact, as my chest hair grew back, one might even miss it.

Unfortunately, because of Dr. Reardon's busy schedule this day, he was too busy to talk with Carole. However, Carole was informed of the results. A sliver of hope emerged that I might finally be out of life-threatening danger.

CHAPTER 2: Aorta Damage

I had never heard about an aortic dissection before, and I had no idea what it was. What I've learned since is that the aorta wall is made up of three layers – the intima, the media, and the externa. My aorta aneurysm had stretched my aorta until a tear in the inner aorta wall (the intima) began. From there, blood pushed in between the layers of the aorta wall, separating the layers. This is a dissection. This had to be that tearing sensation I felt when it happened.

My dissection started near the aorta root, close to the heart, and continued up the ascending aorta to the aortic arch. A dissection in this part of the aorta is called Type A and it is the most dangerous. My dissection continued through the aortic arch, down the descending thoracic aorta, down the abdominal aorta and into my right iliac artery. A dissection in the descending part of the aorta is called Type B.

I also have something called a false lumen in my descending aorta that goes to my right iliac artery. A true lumen is the normal tubular conduit for blood to flow through the aorta. A false lumen is the dissected pathway between the aorta wall layers, resulting from the tear in the wall. My false lumen is patent, or open, meaning that blood is still flowing through it. In fact, my false lumen is supplying blood to my right iliac artery. The disadvantage with this is that the blood pressure in the false lumen can sometimes push down onto the true lumen, restricting its blood flow. Luckily, I am not affected by this.

~~~~~~~~~~~~~

As far as what caused my dissection, there was no clear answer. Something had to have weakened my aortic wall. There are a variety of possible reasons. For some people, it is due to a connective tissue disorder, like Marfan Syndrome or Ehlers-Danlos Syndrome. For others, it could be due to having a congenital defect or after having had an injury. Then there are some that get it from having uncontrolled, chronic high blood pressure, including participating in high-intensity activities such as heavy weightlifting. Still, there are other means.

One of those other means is the usage of a class of antibiotics called fluoroquinolones, like Levaquin. These antibiotics are extremely strong and have been found that they could weaken the aortic wall. I have taken this type of antibiotics at least a half dozen times. Ruling out the usual causes, my personal belief is that this is how I contracted this condition.

At the time I took these antibiotics, there was no written side effect about a possible aortic weakening. However, since my dissection, these antibiotics now list aortic dissection as a possible side effect.

So, much later, after my recovery, I contacted a lawyer to see if I might have a lawsuit against the drug company that manufactured this antibiotic.

What I found out is that since I had taken the generic form of the drug, I could not sue. This all stems back to a Supreme Court ruling on generic drug companies. Apparently, generic drug companies are required by federal regulations to post the same drug information as the brand-name company. This means that generic drug companies cannot be held liable concerning the drug information, since they are beholden to the brand-name company. But what's ridiculous is that
~~~~~~~~~~~~~

I am also not able to sue the brand-name company either, since they weren't the ones who actually manufactured the drug I took. In this case, consumer be damned, especially since more and more prescription companies are forcing members to take generic drugs.

CHAPTER 3: Dream?

I awaken. I'm in the operating room lying on a table. The room is gloomy. It seems dark, an unsettling gray. I don't hear anything, but I sense the doctor nearby. Then, suddenly, I feel like I'm floating above the table. I realize that my body has just died, but my spirit remains. I desperately try to return to my body, but I cannot will myself to do so. I sense the doctor saying I have died, and he has already tried multiple times to save me. I fear that the doctor has given up on me.

Now I sense Carole nearby. She's upset, frantic, even angry. She demands that the doctor try again. Now, Tobie is there too. But Tobie walks away, thinking Carole is fighting a losing battle. Carole refuses to leave. I struggle with all my will to remain, to survive and be with my wife. I struggle to give some indication that I'm still here before the doctor leaves. However, I sense the table being rolled away, and I fear that I will be forever gone, lost to this world, but more importantly, lost to Carole. I feel my spirit, my soul, draining away. I've never been so scared.

CHAPTER 4: ICU

I had never been in an ICU before. Nor had I ever been admitted to a hospital other than for outpatient services. So, the following experience was all new to me.

~~~~~~~~~~~~~

My stay began with me being unconscious. Besides being sedated due to the surgery and intubation, my body had just been through hell and needed time to rest. But even though I was not awake, the doctors still ran plenty of tests, and the nurses were still quite busy tending to me. I was just not aware of any of this. Carole was, however, and she was quite worried about my critical state.

Carole came and left over the next few days, watching me lie there in bed, not moving, wondering how long it would take before I finally woke, fearful that I never would. Not knowing what to expect, Carole asked Dr. Reardon about my unconscious state, trying to ascertain how I was doing. He stressed to her to not be surprised if I didn't wake up right away, that it could take up to one, even two weeks. Much depended upon when my body sensed that I had healed enough. That didn't alleviate Carole's worry much, and it wouldn't for as long as I remained unconscious. So, as I lay there, under sedation, Carole's fear had her constantly questioning if I
~~~~~~~~~~~~~

would survive this. After all, what I just went through was extremely traumatic for both of us.

~~~~~~~~~~~~~

After three days, the nurses tried to wake me by reducing my sedation. They checked how I responded, especially my breathing. It was time to try to wean me off the ventilator, but first they needed to see if my oxygen levels were okay. When I did finally start to wake, my thoughts were cloudy. I saw that I was in some huge room, but I didn't realize yet it was a hospital ICU.

My only memory was a disturbing one – a vivid memory of dying in the operating room. To me, it was real. So, based on my dream, I thought that I was actually dead. Was this the afterlife? I felt lost and began wondering, what could I do? My first thought was to somehow get to Carole. But how? I didn't know where I was, or if it was even possible to get to Carole. That's when the fear set in. What if I never saw Carole again? Again, thinking that I was truly dead, I began thinking that I could just will my spirit to float around and look for something I could recognize. If I could just make it to Carole, maybe I could show her that I wasn't gone.

I began drifting off to sleep once more...

~~~~~~~~~~~~~

I woke again. This time, a nurse was telling me that I was in the hospital. I wasn't sure what to believe. A part of me, a large part, still thought I was dead.

I was too drowsy to think...

~~~~~~~~~~~~~

I came to once more. This time, Carole and Jennifer were there. My mind was really fuzzy. I finally realized that I was in the hospital, but I didn't understand what was going on. I had no clue as to why I
~~~~~~~~~~~~~

was here. Nor did I care. Even when Carole held and squeezed my hand for support and love, I didn't fully realize it. She then asked if it was okay if Jennifer squeezed my hand. I didn't want to, though to this day I have no idea why I did that. All I can say now is that my mind was not right yet.

I felt very relaxed except for there being something stuck in my throat. I needed to get whatever it was out. I didn't understand that it was my breathing tube. I did remember trying to lift my arms to reach my mouth. I strained with all my might to move my hand towards my mouth, but something kept me from doing so. Why couldn't I lift my arms? Carole told me later that my arms had been restrained. It was not unexpected for patients to try to pull out their breathing tube.

As I tried to move my arms, Carole noticed that my right arm was having problems. Later, I heard someone asking me to lift my arms. Apparently, I was having trouble with one of my arms. But being barely awake, I didn't care.

I just wanted to go back to sleep...

~~~~~~~~~~

It was now Saturday night, over four days of being sedated. I woke again. This time, I was a little more conscious. Thankfully, the nurse said I could get this damn tube out of my throat. After telling me to take a deep breath, she pulled it out. Surprisingly, I didn't gag as much as I would have expected. I felt a small sense of relief. I don't remember much else.

~~~~~~~~~~

It was very late on the same night after having my breathing tube extubated. Jennifer was still awake at our house and decided to call the ER to check if I had fully awakened yet. They informed her that I had, and even though it was off hours, they told her that she could talk with me if she wanted to. Jennifer went to wake Carole and tell her the good news.

It was about 3:00 a.m. when I finally talked with Carole and Jennifer on the phone. At least that was what Carole later told me. I have only a vague recollection of the event. Obviously, Carole was ecstatic that I was finally awake, but for some reason I told her, "It isn't over yet." To this day, I have no idea why I said that. Maybe it was from the medications. Maybe it was because I still thought I was dead, and I wasn't sure if I was really talking with Carole. I wasn't sure what was real.

~~~~~~~~~~

It was now day five of my event, Sunday morning. I was awake, but I was still mentally out of it. What was funny was that I was not scared, anxious, or concerned. Probably due to all the medications I was on, but also probably due to all the trauma I went through. Of course, I still didn't know what happened to me. I didn't know that I cheated death. I had no idea why I was in the hospital. I would not learn that until much later.

So, for the most part, I would strangely find the ICU very comforting, even relaxing. And, except for when I had visits from Carole or my doctors, or when I had medical tests or medications given to me, I had nothing to do but lie there and rest. So, I spent my time observing. I watched the nurses. I watched the doctors. I watched those patients within my view, even though most seemed to be unconscious. And I tried to listen to the conversations around me. There were many stories to be heard. It was all very entertaining. At least to me in my fuzzy state of mind.

A Brief Scare

When it came time again for the morning visiting hours, Carole and Jennifer returned to the ICU, eager to talk with me now that I was awake. However, when they went in, they saw that my spot in the ICU room was vacant, and they didn't know where I was. With a
~~~~~~~~~~

twist of bad humor, Jennifer overheard a nurse saying that someone coded during the night. With not seeing me, she immediately wondered if it was me that coded. She was afraid that the worst had happened, that I had died. She wasn't sure what to do or say. What Carole and Jennifer soon discovered, thank God, was that I had been moved to another location in the same ICU room. Jennifer told Carole later what she overheard, and how it scared the hell out of her.

Visiting Hours

Even though I wouldn't remember everything in the first couple of days of my being awake, I did remember relishing the times when Carole and Jennifer came to visit. Note that I still did not fully believe Carole and Jennifer were real, and that somehow, I was just imagining all of this. Regardless, they did cheer me up, and I looked forward to the moments in the day when they were allowed in. The only problem was that visiting hours weren't very long in the critical ICU. The good news was that I had no real conception of time, so time passed by quickly.

Teaching Hospital

Houston Methodist Hospital at the Texas Medical Center is a teaching hospital. So, it wasn't surprising to find residents accompanying the doctors on their rounds. The first time this happened while Carole was in the ICU, she was told that she could ask the residents anything. Taking advantage of that, Carole asked them, what were my chances of recovery? They told her that they knew of no reason why I shouldn't be able to have a full recovery. That made her feel much better. Even though it wasn't her favorite thing to do, asking questions would be something she had to do for days to come. It was just one example of her inner strength, something I admire her for.

Carole's Strength

Being consumed by my ordeal, and still not thinking clearly, I didn't realize the turmoil that Carole was going through. Looking back now at how Carole presented such a calm face to me whenever she visited, I am thoroughly impressed by her strength, strength she thought she never had. I definitely believe that God gave her the strength to handle such a dire situation. I say this because, normally, anxiety and Carole are good friends, which would have made this whole mess quite an ordeal for her.

Carole would wait till I was much better before telling me of some of what she had to endure – making an hour drive to and from the hospital every day for three weeks straight (and during Houston rush hour traffic), working with all the doctors and staff to handle all of my medical care, working with my employer on putting me on short-term disability, taking care of everything at our home, taking care of all the bills, which I normally do, and the biggest stressor – dealing with the fact that I almost died (twice) and still not knowing what would be the extent of my final condition (assuming that nothing else happened to me).

I don't know if I could have been as strong if the situation was reversed. I only knew that during my recovery, in my limited awareness, Carole was providing me a ray of hope and gave me motivation to keep moving forward. I feel bad now that I didn't alleviate some of her worries. But again, I wasn't lucid yet. So, in some ways, I was having a much easier time than her. At least for early on.

All Hooked Up

I didn't really think about what was going on in the ICU. It was as if this was all normal. In fact, what was really weird was I didn't really think about why I was here. I just accepted it. I was probably still in shock. Or maybe it was the medications. Regardless, I just went along with whatever the doctors and nurses did with me, including giving me all sorts of medications, and hooking me up to all sorts of equipment.

Earlier, when I was still unconscious, Jennifer's husband, Scott, took a picture of me all hooked up. At first, Carole was upset with this, thinking it was not right to do. But later, she asked for a copy of the picture, thinking it would be an interesting keepsake. I would not look at this picture until several weeks later because it was too emotional to see myself so close to death. When I finally did take a look, it was disconcerting to see the sign over me stating "Open Chest," plus seeing the large amount of medical equipment attached to me.

I had at least one IV connected to countless drips, a central line in my neck, a chest tube for drainage, a catheter going to a urine bag, a feeding line running through my nose and down my throat, and heart monitor leads on my chest. (As far as the chest tube, thank God I was unconscious when they pulled it out. I've been told that it is very painful when pulled out.)

Awake and lying in bed, I could see and hear all sorts of equipment in the room, those hooked up to me as well as those hooked up to other patients. To this day, hearing sounds similar to this equipment instantly brings me back to being in the ICU, especially that consistent beeping of the monitors, or the noise that the IV drips make when they run out of medication. Oh, how those sounds in the ICU gave me an eerie feeling. Not a scary feeling, more of a soothing memory, almost a fondness. Remember, I was still not really aware of my predicament, so being in the ICU was not a bad thing. Isn't that ridiculous?

Also, looking around the room, I could see a few other patients, some conscious, some not. There were a couple of patients with even more equipment hooked up to them than me. It may have been my delirium, but I counted over thirty hookups on one patient. Carole told me that I was probably right, though. I didn't know it at the time, but this particular ICU room of about six patients was for the most critical. Lucky me.

ICU Delirium

Speaking of delirium, that was something else that I never experienced or heard of before – ICU delirium. Apparently, it was a combination of the pain medicines, the trauma of the situation, the disruption of normal sleep, and the lights and noise of the ICU causing one to hallucinate. As real as I see and hear things today, I could have sworn that all of the things I saw and heard in the ICU were real. But as I would find out later, not everything I remembered was trustworthy.

For some reason, one of my more common hallucinations was that I kept hearing instrumental music while watching psychedelic colors and patterns flash and swirl around me on the walls and ceiling. It was all very enjoyable, and it kept me entertained. However, in my delirious state, I for some reason became afraid that the nurses and other patients in the ICU were starting to blame me for the disruption caused by these lights and noise (after all, it was an ICU and people were trying to rest). So, I began thinking that I was causing the colors and music to happen. Somehow, from my death experience, I had gained "powers." What was even more comical was that I began to try to act like I didn't notice the noise and disco lights, hoping that people wouldn't think it was me doing it.

Then, there were the conversations that I thought I heard. Like the doctor saying that I was given a special type of heart valve, extracted from some type of sea creature, a mermaid, even. Or, that my surgery was so groundbreaking that Dr. Reardon and I were going to be in the news.

But the worst part of my delirium was one night when I thought my nurses were trying to kill me, and I begged for mercy. They finally sedated me (not sure if it was due to all of my whining or not), and at the time, I thought this was it, that they were giving me a lethal injection. I watched them look at me with this evil, sadistic grin as they put the needle into my IV. Or at least that's what my delirium saw. I remembered feeling a sense of sadness that I survived my ordeal only to be murdered. And why would they murder me? Because of all the disturbance I was causing with that damn music and light show.

Anyway, I did not get murdered, and my nurses were, in fact, quite wonderful. And the delirium would only last for a few days. However, to this day, I miss hearing the music and seeing the psychedelic colors. That was quite special, and a bit comforting.

Dreams of Red

There were other things that were not so comforting. After several days of being sedated, I would find it hard to go back to sleep. But it was not because I did not get tired. For days after, whenever I shut my eyes, I saw nothing but waves of dark red – *blood* red. These waves of blood washed over any visions in my head. Everything was painted by this deep red.

No matter how hard I tried, I could not change the disturbing images. It scared me. It may have been the delirium, or it may have been haunting visions from an unconscious mind somehow aware of the bloody trauma that my body went through in surgery. Regardless, I would not sleep again for the remainder of my time in ICU.

Swallowing

I'm sure it was the strong medications given to me, but I was not in any pain. My only torment was a severe dry throat. It's what I would think being stranded in a desert for a week would feel like. So, it was natural that I was thirsty.

Not long after I was fully awake, the nurse tried to give me a sip of water, but I immediately choked on it. I discovered that I could not swallow. My throat muscles would not work. It was attributed to my throat muscles being atrophied after being on a breathing tube for four and a half days.

Luckily, the central line inserted into my throat allowed the nurse to give me certain medications. And, whenever the nurse injected a medicine through this line, I relished the cool liquid on the back of my throat. It would be the only satisfying quench for me until weeks later.

Craving something to drink, I told Carole that an ice-cold beer would be nice. But, since that obviously couldn't happen, I would settle for some very cold apple juice. Unfortunately, nothing could be given to me to drink. So, in the meantime, all I could have to satisfy my dry mouth were moist swabs and an occasional very small ice cube. Even though I desperately wanted to try again, the doctors were scared that I would aspirate and risk getting pneumonia.

Kidneys

One issue that I didn't even think about, but Carole sure did was – how were my kidneys? At the time, I had Stage III Chronic Kidney Disease due to IgA Nephropathy. It had been a slow, progressive disease for me – for over twenty-five years. While I was still sedated, Carole worried that my kidneys might have been damaged. Apparently, my kidney functions got really bad (my serum creatinine jumped from 2.0 to 3.6).

At first, Methodist Hospital had one of their nephrologists come in, but Carole demanded that they contact my regular nephrologist instead – Dr. Rajeev Raghavan from Baylor College of Medicine. Dr. Raghavan was notified of my situation, and he sent over one of his colleagues, Dr. Yan, to check on me. When Dr. Yan got there, she eased Carole's worry, stating that the fact that I was still putting out any urine at all was a good sign. She also told Carole not to be too concerned about my kidney functions for now, that though my kidneys were damaged (or *insulted,* as they call it), she expected that they would improve in time. Of course, a concern with aorta dissections, though, is that it could lead to a loss of blood to the kidneys and severely damage them, even causing them to go into complete failure. Luckily, mine would not. However, my trauma did cause some temporary kidney damage. How much and whether permanent was yet to be seen.

Bedpan

My only other noteworthy time in ICU concerned the use of a bedpan. This was a first for me. I always thought that I could never go to the bathroom using a bedpan, but that was before surviving death.

Being in ICU, I could not use a bathroom. So, when it finally came time for me to go, the nurse helped me to a chair next to my bed, gave me a bedpan, closed some curtains around me, and helped me sit on the bedpan (note that I was too weak and unsteady to do this on my own). So, there I was, sitting and trying to go, with several people around me in the ICU, with nothing but a flimsy sheet between me and people only a few feet away. But this wasn't the worst of it.

Once I finished my business, I could not wipe myself due to the weakness in my right arm and hand. My nurse had to do that for me. *And it was a male nurse.* It must had been my current mental state (or medications), but I was not that embarrassed.

I was very grateful to my nurse. Besides the lifesaving care these nurses performed, they were wonderful in how they treated their patients. I was thoroughly impressed at my nurse's professionalism in handling such a private and sensitive matter. Kudos to all nurses.

Minor Strokes

Of the next couple of days I spent in this ICU room, I had several more tests performed, including many EKGs and ultrasounds. Besides checking out my heart and my aorta, the doctors were also checking into why I had weakness in my right arm (they were also concerned that some of my delirium may have been brain related). I didn't know it at the time (or at least I didn't remember anything being said), but the doctors were concerned that I may have had a stroke. Carole knew about this, and she was deeply concerned. She was initially afraid when I couldn't raise my right arm after the first time I awoke, but then I was also slurring my speech. Again, I was not too coherent, and I didn't recognize any adverse speech problems. So, the neurologist assigned to me, Dr. Thomas, ordered an MRI of my head and an MRA of my neck.

First of all, note that I am extremely claustrophobic. So, I was very concerned about being put into the MRI machine. However, still on some good drugs, and still in some state of delirium, I was relaxed enough to give it a try. Wheeling me into the MRI room, they proceeded to put me into this very small tube-like contraption. I equated it to a small torpedo tube. They had me lie facedown before securely encasing me. It was so tight that I could not move, even a little. They gave me a squeeze ball to signal to the operator to pull me out, should I get too freaked out. Thinking back on it, I'm amazed that I was able to get into this thing even for a minute, considering that I barely fit into the damn thing. It is not something that I could do now, at least not without being heavily sedated.

As they rolled me into the MRI machine, my face was literally just a couple of inches away from the bottom. I kept thinking about how calm I was at that moment. Then, the loud banging and clicking began. Interestingly enough, the noise was timed to a musical theme, which made it a bit more tolerable (at least I think it was being timed to music; after all, my delirium may have just been entertaining me again). Making absolutely sure I had a hold of the squeeze ball, I tried to remain calm.

After about a half hour or so (it was hard to tell time when you're trying your hardest not to lose it), I started to get panicky. I tried to concentrate on the musical clicking, but all I could think about was being trapped inside this small tube, physically unable to move. I forced myself not to move, because I knew if I tried and couldn't, I would go berserk. Finally, I could no longer stand it and I squeezed the ball. I needed to get out. The operator spoke to me, saying that they were almost done and asked if I could hang on for just another ten minutes. I relented, going back to concentrating on the musical clicking, closing my eyes and trying to concentrate on something else. However, all I could see with my eyes closed were those disturbing waves of red. I was freaking out a little, but I forced myself to comply. After it was done, I was so relieved to get out of that tube. I thanked the operator several times.

What Carole and I learned from the MRI was that I had suffered two minor strokes – one to the right rear cerebellum region and one to the left front parietal vertex of my brain. No one said what caused the strokes, though (from the surgery, from contaminants in the heart/lung bypass machine, from the dissection or something else).

When first told, I didn't know what to think of it. Because currently, I was not thinking of myself as having anything debilitating, at least other than swallowing (which now became unclear if it was due to throat muscle atrophy or my stroke or both). It would not be until later when I started to comprehend that I had issues, that I actually broke down and cried. Carole, on the other hand, was very concerned about what this meant for my recovery – and my long-term outcome. She stayed strong in front of me, but she had her cry later that day after she left.

CHAPTER 5: Out of Critical Care

The next day, Tuesday, one full week now after my event, someone came around to get me up out of bed. They wanted to see if I could walk. With help, I could, though only by hanging onto the person and taking baby steps. Plus, they only had me walk down a short corridor and back. I must have done well enough because they told me that I was getting better. In response, they prepared to send me to a less intensive ICU. I guess I was *graduating*.

~~~~~~~~~~~~

It would not be until nighttime before I was moved. So, as I was rolled into my new ICU room, the room was already dark, making it hard to see what the room looked like, or what was even in there. I knew that there were other patients there, sleeping, but I could barely see them. I began feeling uneasy. This ICU did not *feel* like the critical care ICU, and that feeling would begin to play on my mind. For when they settled me into my new spot, I had it in my mind that they just abandoned me in some random open spot. It was obvious, at least to me, that I was not going to be as closely monitored in here. But as will be seen, part of my uneasiness may have been that my delirium was still active.

As I lay there, with my eyes adjusting to the dim light, I began to take in my new surroundings. In my deceptive mind, it appeared as if the center of the room was filled with tables for tea and food, sort of a
~~~~~~~~~~~~

café area. Plus, I was hearing jungle noises in the background. For some reason, that made me think that they were trying to make the place be like Vietnam. I couldn't imagine why I would have thought of that, especially since I had never been to Vietnam. Sitting at the tables were people eating and drinking. They appeared to be Asian. Vietnamese? I thought so, in my delirium. I assumed they were nurses, but I wasn't sure. However, the experience (or I should say my delusion) was strangely soothing. At least I found some entertainment.

When I woke the next day, none of my delusions about the room remained. No café. Not Vietnam. My bed wasn't left out in the open. I was in a normal ICU room. However, I would quickly discover that I didn't care much to be in this room, for two reasons. There was not as much activity (or interest) in this room as there had been with all of the constant attention required in critical care, and the head nurse in this room was not nearly as caring. Or, I should say she was not as caring about her patients. She was *caring* about talking with the male members of the hospital staff. Fortunately, I would stay in this ICU room for only about a day until I could get transferred to a standard patient room.

And there seemed to be a mutual feeling of dislike with the head nurse. I wasn't sure what I did to provoke her (besides trying to sit up on my bed every now and then), but in response to my unrest, she told Carole that I was going to be a handful. Which, considering the fact that I was just diagnosed with two strokes, caused Carole to fear that I might have more severe problems than she knew about. That remark from the nurse really scared Carole. Luckily, that nurse's prediction would not turn out to be true (at least not to the extent she insinuated). In response to the nurse's insensitive remark, my stepdaughter, Jennifer, reported the nurse for her thoughtlessness. Never heard if she got in trouble or not.

But because of my eagerness (or stubbornness, depending on who you asked) to move around, Carole was told that I could not be moved to a standard room unless there would be someone there to watch over me at all times. In other words, I needed a babysitter. They were afraid that I would try to get out of bed and fall. I guess I was not regarded as being trustworthy. Because of this and other behavior of mine, I would eventually learn that my personality had changed somewhat. The question was, was it due to my medications, my strokes, or my PTSD from nearly dying?

Standard Patient Room

In order to get me to a standard patient room, Carole had the hospital assign me a hospital aide, to be in my room for whenever Carole was not there. Again, this was due to that trust issue (or lack of). Regardless, I was finally brought to a private room, and I was glad to discover that I was in a private room.

Being out of ICU, Carole and I were much happier. Beside meaning that I was one step closer to recovery, she could spend much more time with me instead of the very short ICU visiting hours. In addition, having now been out of critical care for a day or so, my delirium was starting to wear off, and I was becoming more alert. The only downside was that I still missed all of the action in ICU.

In all, I would spend about seven days in this room.

Taking Vitals

Taking vitals – a constant ritual. It started back on my first day in ICU, and it would continue for my entire hospital stay. Blood pressure, temperature, and blood sugar. For some reason, maybe the medications they gave me, they were concerned with my blood sugar. So, I got my fingers pricked all the time, sometimes ten or more times a day. My poor fingertips. After a while, I started getting used to it.

And it was just like the jokes about being in the hospital. You had no time to rest as they regularly came in to check on you. But I didn't really mind. Except for maybe during the night. Regardless, the vast majority of my nurses were extremely nice, and they were a welcomed distraction.

Blood Thinners

One thing I did not like from my nurses' visits was when it was time for my blood thinner injection. Because of the major cardiac surgery I had, and since I was still pretty much immobile, I needed a heavy-duty blood thinner to prevent blood clots. That called for Heparin injections. And Heparin injections are usually given in the abdomen. Why the abdomen? Well, I didn't know why at the time, and it never occurred to me to ask back then, even when I cringed as they injected me, but I found out later that Heparin injections must be given subcutaneously into fatty tissue. The most common site is the abdominal fat pad due to ease of access. Anyway, this was a first for me to get shots in my stomach. Luckily, the needle was not too big, and it didn't hurt much. It was more of a mental thing.

A-fib

As in ICU, I was still hooked up to a heart monitor. At some point, I was told that I had gone into Atrial Fibrillation (A-fib), a quivering, irregular heartbeat. Some of the times, I could even feel it. It was a little disturbing to feel your heart quiver like that, and even worse when it continued for several seconds or more.

Apparently, it was not uncommon to have A-fib after heart surgery. The trauma from such surgery "angers" the heart. Of course, this brought about more tests to ensure that I was stable. My A-fib would happen off and on for the near term and would remain a concern even till today.

Vision Problems

Now that I was getting better, it was time for me to regain some stamina for walking. Carole, and sometimes the hospital rehab staff, would help me walk around the corridors. I was still too unsteady to walk without someone to hold onto, but I was getting around, albeit very slowly.

However, now that I was up and about, I began noticing that I was having trouble with my vision. Looking down while walking got me really dizzy. In addition, when I tried to look up, it was hard to initially gain focus. I had to really concentrate on gaining focus, as if my eyes had become wobbly. And what was strange, it was only when changing my vision from looking down to looking up. Any other change in direction seemed okay. It was all rather disorienting, and it really concerned me. I didn't know if this was weakness from the surgery, something related to my stroke, my medicines, or something else completely. No one else knew either.

[*To this day, I still experience this problem, though my brain seems to have adapted to it, lessening the intensity of the disorientation. More on my vision later.*]

Besides my focusing issue, Carole also noticed that my eyes did not track with my head movements, especially when talking with people. I would be looking in one direction, and when I turned my head to look elsewhere, my eyes didn't follow in a timely manner, and sometimes appeared as if I wasn't looking straight at the person. I didn't notice anything myself. Another oddity to be resolved.

Rehab

Now that I was improving, I had thought that it wouldn't be too long before I got to a point where I could be sent home. But another doctor came in to help Carole decide what local hospital to transfer me to where I could undergo rehab. Rehab? Up until now, no one had mentioned that my road to recovery would be a long one.

The doctor talked more with Carole than me, which was a good thing since I wasn't sure why I even needed rehab. I was thinking that all I needed to do was gain a little more strength so I could move around on my own. Now they were talking about me needing different therapies. I just didn't know what therapies they thought I needed, though. I also understood them to say that I would still need medical monitoring, which the rehab hospital would also provide. So, if I needed medical monitoring, why transfer me to a rehab hospital and not stay where I was? Couldn't they do rehab here? Well, as I was told later, a rehab hospital provided therapies for stabilized patients at a reduced cost than a regular hospital. So, this was about money and hospital resources.

Unfortunately, this became yet another item that Carole had to take upon herself for me. I was so glad she was here to help.

Bathroom

Another bright spot being out of ICU was that I was allowed to use a regular bathroom. The only downside was that I had to have someone in the bathroom with me to watch over me, to help me in and out and to make sure I did not fall. I didn't like this requirement, but I understood why it was needed. I was glad when my nurse relented and allowed Carole to help me instead. Actually, I was adamant (a nicer way of saying stubborn) that I wanted Carole instead of the nurse to go in with me. But even that was a bit embarrassing as I had never had someone be with me when I had to have a bowel movement. Even after nearly thirty years of marriage.

[*This intolerable attitude of mine was just the beginning, as I would find out in months to come. It was an attitude that concerned Carole. She would begin reading up on stroke victim behavior. Something I would not want to hear.*]

When I finally used the bathroom, I discovered that my stool was black. Carole called in the nurse for her to see, worried that it might have been blood. However, my nurse chalked it up to the iron they were giving me since I am so anemic. I would soon find out that this was not the case. Even though the nurse was a very nice person, this was a major mistake on her part.

Feeding Tube

The most debilitating issue I was still facing was the fact that I could not swallow, and therefore I could not eat or drink. Each time I tried, I choked. So, my only nutrition came in the form of a liquid diet via a nasal line and IVs.

For the most part, the feeding tube had not been a hindrance. However, one night while becoming restless, I became fed up with the irritation of the nasal line. The line just seemed to be getting in my way as I tossed and turned. Maybe it was because I was getting more alert, but the damn thing was really bothering me. So, when the line got snagged once again, and this time got partially pulled out, I figured why not pull out the rest of it. And I did. Half asleep, I didn't realize that the line was still dripping food on my bed. I just left the line by my side and tried to get some sleep, which I finally did.

The next day, the nursing staff was not too happy with my antics. They wouldn't put another nasal line in me. I didn't know if it was because of a medical reason, that they didn't trust me to leave another line in, or if they were merely irritated with me. So, instead of a feeding line, they hooked me up to an IV diet of sucrose for the next couple of days.

By the time I would get home from the hospital, I had lost eighteen pounds, going from 158 to 140 pounds. Which wasn't too bad a thing when I saw myself in the mirror. My stomach hadn't been that flat in years. So, when I talked with other people later, I told them that it was good to be a little overweight. Just in case you ended up in the hospital on a liquid diet.

Forcing the situation now, Carole and I asked to see an ENT doctor about examining my throat to see why I could not swallow. It took a couple of days, but an ENT doctor finally showed up. One test I was given was to x-ray my throat as they watched me try to swallow. That wouldn't be successful as I immediately gagged. Because of the dismal result, they said that I would need to give it more time before I could try again. Until then, I was back to only ice chunks to chew on, and NO SWALLOWING! Frustrated, I still tried to swallow a minute sip of the melted ice every now and then, which made me cough. But that brought instant consternation from my nurses. They threatened to not give me any more ice unless I obeyed. I reluctantly agreed to their demands. But could I help it if there happened to be a little too much water in my mouth every now and then?

Since I was nearing my time to be released to a rehab hospital, and since it appeared that I wouldn't be swallowing anytime soon, the subject of a Percutaneous Endoscopic Gastronomy (PEG) feeding tube came up, because staying just on an IV for nutrients long-term would not do. For some reason, being put on a feeding tube didn't bother me. And, since I couldn't leave the hospital until I got one, I looked forward to getting one as soon as possible. Probably not too many people can say that. However, it would take them another two days before they finally scheduled me to have a PEG feeding tube surgically implanted into my stomach. I didn't know why it took them so long.

It was now Friday, and the surgery went without issue. They basically cut a hole into my stomach and inserted a tube with a disc-like mechanism near one end to keep it from being pulled out accidentally. A section of the tube then extended on the outside of my body. At the end of this outer tube is a valve that allowed a large syringe to be connected and deliver liquid food. I was in no pain from the surgery, but I had to be careful of pulling on the external tube.

I would eat, drink, and take my medicines using this tube for several weeks. It was kind of weird, though, having my nurses feed me through this tube. It wasn't that I felt the food going into my stomach, it was just odd to be fed manually. Of course, the nurses were very good about it, and they taught me how to do it myself (which would come in handy sooner than I thought it needed to). And the strange thing was, I never felt hungry or had a craving for food. But, wanting something cold to drink –That was another story.

CHAPTER 6: Rehab Hospital

It was now Monday, August 15th. After a total of fourteen days at Methodist Hospital, I was finally released to a rehab hospital, the supposedly next step in my recovery. I was transferred to Kindred Hospital in Clear Lake by ambulance. This ride I would remember, but it was vaguely boring. Which was a good thing.

When I got to Kindred Hospital, they put me straight into a large patient room and left me. I didn't know if this was a private room or just that I was the only one currently in there. Carole came in soon after.

Unfortunately, the nurse assigned to me was brand new. So new, in fact, that she didn't even know how to feed me through my PEG tube when it came time for my feeding. I actually had to step her through it. Made me feel a bit superior. But it also concerned the hell out of Carole and me. Just how new was this nurse? I wasn't really feeling the quality of care that I received at Methodist.

Eventually, with it getting late in the day, and appearing that I was settled in, Carole decided to head home. It was hoped that being close to home (about twenty minutes away) would finally ease some of the burden on Carole. As I would later think about it, she must have been much more exhausted than I was. But, as I said before, I was just beginning to realize my situation. I feel guilty now that I wasn't as concerned as I should have been back then about her welfare.

So, with Carole gone and thinking that I was past the critical stage in my recovery, I tried to relax and hope for the best. I didn't know how long I would be here at Kindred Hospital, and I wasn't even sure what it was that I would be doing here other than recuperating. Regardless, I kept thinking that in maybe a week or so, I would finally be back at home. However, I was also thinking that my care here at Kindred would be similar to my previous care at Methodist Hospital. Boy, was I wrong on that last thought.

Another Emergency

Not long after Carole left to go home, I began feeling pain in my left arm. Not thinking much about it, I called for a nurse for some painkiller, just like I used to do at Methodist Hospital. But the nurses were in the midst of a shift change. I was told that someone would be in shortly. Minutes went by and the pain was getting worse. I called for a nurse again, and I was told again that my nurse would be in as soon as she could, but I would have to wait. Well, time kept flowing and still no nurse. It seemed like several minutes now and no one had stepped into my room to see what was going on with me. This was nothing like the care at Methodist Hospital, and, quite frankly, very irresponsible to me.

It didn't take much longer before my pain level rose to excruciating. This was ridiculous. Here I am in severe pain, in a hospital, and I can't get anyone to come check on me. I couldn't take it anymore. So, all I could think of was to call Carole and tell her about what was going on. Distressed beyond my breaking point, I told her that if she didn't come and get me soon, that I would call an ambulance myself to get me out of this damn place. Poor Carole didn't know what to do, so she called our friend, Allyson, to go with her back to Kindred Hospital.

Before Carole and Allyson arrived, I sat myself down on the floor and leaned against my bed in agony. I'm not sure why I did this other than it felt good to do so. A nurse finally came in and saw me on the floor. Finally concerned over my well-being, the nurse called for others, including the doctor. At first, they assumed that I had fallen, but I told them that I purposely got to the floor, trying to find some relief from my pain. I told them that I was in severe pain.

Soon, Carole and Allyson arrived, and they tried to assess what was going on. As when I originally dissected, my memory got a bit fuzzy again. Was it due to the pain or something else? I didn't know.

To see what might be causing my pain, the doctor had ordered some blood work. What they discovered was that my hemoglobin had gotten down to about five mg (thirteen is the low limit). I was bleeding somewhere and the pain in my arm was due to a lack of blood, just like with my leg from my dissection.

Since Kindred Hospital was for rehab and not emergency care, I could not be treated here. I was told that an ambulance was called to take me to the emergency room at another hospital. Whatever they decided to do was fine with me, because all I cared about right now was to have someone give me some damn pain medication. Plus, I wanted away from this hospital.

CHAPTER 7: Back to Methodist

When the ambulance arrived, the ambulance personnel first checked on the availability of a nearby hospital. They were told that they could not take me there. Didn't know why. So, instead, they took me back to St. John Hospital. Which was fine with me, because I trusted them.

At St. John Hospital, it took a while to be treated, and I again had to suffer in agony. Also, like the last time, I repeatedly begged for pain medication. Why wouldn't they give me something for the pain? After about two hours, instead of pain medication, they finally gave me a pint of blood. It *slowly* began to help. I tried to calm myself as I waited for relief. It took a long time, at least to someone in pain.

They also informed me that they would be transferring me back to Houston Methodist Hospital, because that was where I could receive the best care, considering my dissection. And since it was now very late at night, and since I had finally stabilized, Carole told me that she would not be following me there. It would do her no good. Plus, she was exhausted. Instead, she went home to get some much-needed rest before having to drive all the way back to Methodist – once again! So much for things getting easier for her. And there I was – once again – not considering the turmoil she was going through. I would make it up to her later, but just one more reason for me to feel guilty later.

So, another ambulance ride. On the way, they gave a bag of frozen blood plasma for additional support. By the time I got to Methodist Hospital, I was feeling much better.

Bleeding Ulcer

I was back in an ICU, but not the critical care ICU like I was in before. Dr. Fan was the ICU doctor on staff, and he would be the one who took charge of my admittance this time. Since he saw that I was stable, he decided to wait until the next morning before running any tests. Besides no longer being in pain, being back at Methodist Hospital calmed me. I felt safe here. I knew that I was properly being monitored.

Come morning, Carole was there. And, as she had been all along, she remained strong in front of me. What a wonderful wife!

To confirm the source of my bleeding, Dr. Peter Schwarz, a gastroenterologist, was called in to perform an endoscopy. Due to my recently repaired aorta, I had the endoscopy done right where I was in the ICU. Just in case any complications arose. There were several people stirring around me. Not sure how many were doctors. I was more interested in watching them set up the portable endoscopy equipment.

Once ready, they injected me with Propofol, a sedation medicine. I've had Propofol before. It was very good. And quick. I liked it. And even though it would be only for a brief instance, I would remember the momentary relaxed feeling right before going unconscious.

My next memory was waking up, feeling calm. I was told everything went well. From the endoscopy, it turned out that I had developed a bleeding ulcer, which caused my blood loss and extremely low hemoglobin. Luckily, the endoscopy also showed that my bleeding had stopped.

So, what caused my ulcer? It was attributed to the trauma of my surgery, the blood thinners they put me on, and the fact that I had Barrett's esophagus from a hiatal hernia. What I didn't know at the time, but Carole figured out afterward, was that they never put me back on my Omeprazole that I needed to take for my Barrett's esophagus. That would change as they immediately started me on Omeprazole. Another example of why it's good having a loved one watch over you in the hospital.

I would stay about a day and a half in this ICU before being sent to a private room.

Back to a Standard Room

From the ICU, I was sent to a standard patient room again. This time for seven days. Which, at first, was strange since I was previously deemed okay enough to be sent to rehab. But, for some reason, they now wished to run more tests.

In between the tests, I didn't really have much to do. Besides Carole helping me walk down the hospital corridors in order to regain my strength and stamina, the only other task I was given was to use this breathing tube exerciser apparatus, a spirometer, to help me expel any fluids in my lungs so I didn't develop pneumonia. Initially, it was very difficult to breathe hard, especially considering my chest pain. I would work with the spirometer for weeks.

So, with time on my hands, and finally being able to relax (somewhat), I tried to get back to some type of normalcy. I started watching television. The 2016 Summer Olympics were being televised and I watched some of that, trying to keep busy. However, I was not too interested in anything. It was just nice to have something to distract me, though, especially when Carole wasn't there.

Another bit of normalcy. I was finally able to shower. (By the way, the hospital sponge baths are nothing like what's portrayed in the TV shows and movies – it's just a quick wash down.) Of course, showering had its own difficulties. Like wrapping my feeding tube in a large plastic bandage and trying not to get it wet. I also had to sit on a stool to shower since I was still unsteady on my feet. But it was a step closer to getting my life back.

[*It's funny, but I can still remember the smell of that hospital soap. In fact, whenever I return to the hospital as an outpatient, I will smell the soap in their public bathrooms and immediately feel like I'm back in my hospital room. I've heard before how smells can elicit strong memories. This smell certainly does for me.*]

Cardiac Tests

For some reason, being sent back to Houston Methodist Hospital started a whole new set of doctors for me. Carole wasn't happy about this. She wondered why there wasn't a better continuity of care.

Carole found out that Dr. Zoghbi, the cardiologist who originally saw me, was not called in. By chance, one day, she happened to see Dr. Zoghbi in passing, and she told him that I was back in the hospital. Dr. Zoghbi was surprised. He hadn't heard that I was back. Carole was also surprised that Dr. Zoghbi wasn't even notified. Besides being a wonderful cardiologist (chair of the cardiology department for Methodist), he's also a wonderful and caring person. So, Carole asked Dr. Fan to make sure Dr. Zoghbi was assigned as my cardiologist. This was another example of why you need someone looking out for you, and another example of how strong Carole was.

[*An example of Dr. Zoghbi's caring personality. Later, when I was finally at home, he actually called me to discuss how I was doing. To have such a busy and important physician like Dr. Zoghbi take the time to call someone like me was amazing.*]

~~~~~~~~~~~~~
~~~~~~~~~~~~~

During the rest of my stay, I would be given several cardiac tests. I didn't know why the doctors were currently concerned about my heart after having previously released me. Maybe it was just the new round of doctors. Regardless, one of my tests suggested that I might have some cardiac blockage. That brought even more tests, some of which were quite interesting.

One of the tests was a Cardiac Computerized Tomography (CT) Coronary Angiography that had me lie flat for what seemed like hours. They had me watch a video of outdoors scenes to relax me and keep me focused (mainly, to keep me still). The scenes were quite soothing, and I still remember those peaceful moments. In fact, I would often think about those scenes when I tried to relax later. I wish I could have something like those videos at home.

The results from the CTA were mixed. Apparently, my Left Main Artery had fifty percent stenosis (or narrowing of the artery). Everything else seemed to be okay (ignoring my surgery, dissection, and that my true lumen was severely compressed by my false lumen). Because of my fifty percent stenosis though, more tests were needed to see how much an impact I might have had.

Which led to another test that I did not find so soothing – a stress test of my heart. I've had stress tests before and they weren't too bad. But this one didn't use a treadmill to get my heart rate up because even a brisk walk wasn't a good idea right now considering the state my aorta was in from my surgery. Instead, they performed a chemical stress test referred to as a nuclear stress test. And, due to the seriousness of my current condition, I had several people around me for this test. I wasn't scared about the test until I saw all the people. Didn't know how many of them were doctors. But I surmised that if something went wrong, I was in the right place.

I wasn't sure what to expect from this test other than it was supposed to be over quickly. For the moment, they told me to just lie there. When ready, I was injected with a drug called Regadenoson. This drug caused my heart to race instantly. And not just race like having too much caffeine. It felt like I had just run a mile sprint as fast as I could, and my heart was about to burst out of my chest. The experience was very scary, and I didn't know if this was normal or not. I knew I was being closely monitored, so I tried to remain calm. But it was hard to do so. I feared my heart would give out at any moment. Then, after a minute or so (felt much longer), my heart rate started slowing down. Soon after, my heart was normal again. I was hoping that this was it. I hoped that I wouldn't have to repeat the test. Thankfully, it was over.

The good news from my stress test was that it showed no signs of significant blockages. At least, there was no ischemia (or reduced blood flow). The assistant to Dr. Reardon, my cardiac surgeon, informed Carole that the blockage they saw was probably due to some scar tissue in my Left Main Artery from having to detach and reattach my cardiac arteries to my aorta. Carole and I believed that all was good.

Emotions

As I began to recover, I became more cognizant of what had happened to me. For up until now, I had been sort of calm and distant. It was as if I had been watching myself and not actually taking part in the present. I didn't know if it was due to the medications, the trauma, or something else, something more daunting. Maybe it was merely my way of protecting myself. I didn't know. But no matter what, I hadn't been too troubled or fearful of my situation. But now, I began to realize the extent of my near-death experience. Plus, I was starting to assess my new physical limitations, my complications. My emotions began to stir, and they were not good. And Carole? Well, in some ways, she was going through even more hellish emotions.

From learning about my neurologic test results, my inability to swallow, my slurred speech, and my weak arm and hand, I began to truly accept and understand that I suffered two strokes, and that there was a good possibility that I might have real debilitations. I cried. This was my first cry in the hospital other than from pain. Carole was also very concerned, but she still tried to stay strong for me, even though she was terrified on the inside. She worried about whether I would be able to return to work, about what lifestyle changes both of us would suffer, about what care I would need and for how long. Getting past the initial life-and-death struggle, Carole and I were now faced with a new set of obstacles to deal with.

As if sent on cue (maybe my higher power at work?), the hospital's chaplain came in, gave me a rosary, and prayed with me. He told me that God was not done with me yet (a comment I would hear several times since). It was another break in my wall, and I began to cry all over again. These random bouts of crying would continue throughout my recovery and then some. More on that later.

Pain

For me, the pain from the actual surgery itself was surprisingly not that bad. However, there were some serious pains that I had to deal with. The first, and the worst, was the chest pain from coughing. And it was not just an occasional cough that I had to deal with. Because they were concerned about me getting pneumonia, they made me cough regularly to help get up any residual mucus that may have been in my lungs. But, knowing how painful the coughing would be, the hospital gave me this heart pillow. It was a small, red pillow in the shape of a heart. By hugging that pillow tight against my chest, it helped to alleviate some of the pain from coughing. It was still painful, but not quite as bad. Oh, how that heart pillow became my best friend. And based on how painful my coughing was, I was extremely relieved that I didn't have to sneeze until weeks later, long enough into my recovery that it wasn't painful. Considering how hard I usually sneeze, I don't know what would have happened. I probably would have passed out.

The second pain was a constant pain with my back. I kept thinking it was due to lying in bed for such a long period of time, but I was later told it was due to my open-heart surgery. Apparently, when they crack open your ribs, they arch your back up to get better access to the inside of your chest. It was because of this pain that I would continually ask for pain medication because no matter what I did, or how I positioned myself in bed, I could not relieve this pain. So, they decided to give me fentanyl for the pain to help me sleep. Fentanyl was a very relaxing and soothing drug. It made me feel somewhat euphoric. I could see why people get addicted to it. Luckily, I do not have that addiction trait. My only criticism of fentanyl was that it only allowed me to sleep for about two to three hours at a time (which was long in hospital time considering how often they came to take your vitals and blood). So, on a couple of nights, I would have to get multiple dosages. One of my nurses put in a request to get me a fentanyl patch, but the doctor denied that request. I wasn't told why, but I assumed it had to do with the addictive nature of the drug.

Complications

Again, even though I experienced two minor strokes, I didn't exhibit any severe debilitating complications, mainly just some speech and swallowing issues due to tongue weakness. I remember at one time I told Carole that I talked like I was from Brooklyn. Nothing against people from Brooklyn, but it was how I think I sounded. At the time, I found it amusing. I wasn't so sure Carole did. However, it wasn't known yet if my vision problems (dizziness) were due to my strokes. Only time would tell.

A notable complication not stemming from my strokes was some nerve trauma due to where the heart/lung bypass machine was attached. There was an incision scar just above my right pectoral muscle. It was stapled shut. Supposedly, there is a bundle of nerves near this incision point. Some of these nerves were damaged, or at least traumatized. These nerves affected my right shoulder area, arm, and hand. I should note that there are two types of nerves – motor and sensory, and lucky me, I had both types of nerves traumatized.

I had pain and weakness in my right hand. Both were severe. When I finally tried to wash my right hand, it felt like rubbing sandpaper on raw, open skin due to the sensitive nerves. I could barely tolerate the pain. Plus, I could barely do things with my right hand that I had taken for granted, like making a fist, writing, tying my shoes, opening a bottle, or even something more private like wiping myself in the bathroom. Even though I was right-handed, I was forced to use my left hand no matter how awkward. I laughed at how bad my handwriting was. My writing looked like a preschooler. But it was the best I could do since I could not even hold a pen in my right hand. I also noticed numbness around the incision area, as well as a little numbness extending all the way up to the back of my right ear.

Over time, the nerve trauma would lessen. But it took months before the pain in my right hand completely went away, and even longer for the strength in my right hand to fully return. But, even today, my handwriting is still not as good as it was before, and some of the numbness in my right pectoral area still lingers.

All in all, though, I count myself very lucky considering what could have been. I can certainly handle these minor impacts.

Scars

In addition to the numbness in my right shoulder area, my right pectoral muscle was atrophied. It did not work and still doesn't, even as of today. I fear that it never will. It caused a slight lopsided look to my chest, but it's not too bad. My only other physical disfigurements were the scars from my surgeries.

I had the typical long scar down my chest from the sternotomy, but I was surprisingly grateful that my scar did not look bad. Dr. Reardon and his team did an incredible job sewing me back up. I view it now as a battle scar, something to be proud of that I survived. Other scars included the incision from where the heart/lung bypass machine was hooked up, another from where my chest tube was inserted, and another from where my PEG tube was implanted.

These last two scars almost form a nice line with my belly button, giving me the appearance of having three belly buttons.

Again, I'll take these scars any day, given the alternative.

ENT Camera

It was now over a week since I woke up and I still could not swallow. Carole and I asked to be seen again by an ENT doctor to see if anything had changed. I was hoping that there was at least some improvement, something to give me a little hope. For some reason, it took days before the ENT doctor came to see me.

What the ENT doctor did was put a camera up through my nose and down the back of my throat. I gag easily, so this was something very hard for me to do. I found it amazing that I was able to do it. The good news was that no damage was seen to my throat. The bad news was that there was no answer as to why I could not swallow. I was told that I would just have to give it more time.

So, was my swallowing issue due to my stroke? Carole and I were fearful that it might be. I was trying to accept the fact that I would most likely be on a feeding tube for a very long time. I didn't think Carole was too thrilled about that. Of course, neither was I. But I was still in reactive mode and not fully realizing yet what my future held. I was still dealing with current time.

Because of my inability to swallow, I was set up with a company to deliver me feeding tube supplies and food for when I eventually left the hospital. Actually, they worked with Carole on this. I was still more of a bystander when it came to making decisions. Having to make plans for being on a feeding tube long-term kind of solidified the issue, though. Our fear of this being a true impairment was quite real.

Rehab

Surprisingly, I received very little rehab while in the hospital. The most rehab I got was from my own effort when Carole helped me walk. Someone did come to work with me (twice, I think) to show me what minimal exercises I could do for now. Nothing strenuous or hard, just basic movements of my arms and legs. I was shocked, though, not just by the muscle atrophy from being laid up for days, but also the awkwardness of trying to move my body. I was still very weak, but I was also very dizzy and unbalanced.

Besides the physical complications I already mentioned, it was apparent that I would need further rehab just in regard to getting back my physical stamina. That was one of the reasons they sent me to a rehab hospital earlier. However, this time, they were planning on sending me home. Not sure why I got to go directly home now. I guess they thought I was mobile enough to be able to take care of myself. Regardless, I was happy about it, and so was Carole. One of the stipulations, though, was that I would go and get rehab at a facility. That was when the rehab doctor came in.

Stepping into my room one day was Dr. Chan. He said that he had been assigned to work with me on planning my rehab. As with everything else, he actually worked with Carole. Together, Dr. Chan and Carole set me up to go back to the Kindred Hospital, but this time as an outpatient to its rehab facility. I was told that I needed Physical Therapy to condition my body, Speech Therapy to work with my speech and my swallowing (I never realized before that speech and swallowing were interconnected), and Occupational Therapy to regain the use of my right hand. Though it still hadn't quite settled in for me yet, there was a lot of work ahead.

CHAPTER 8: Return Home

It was now August 24th, just over three weeks from my event. It was finally time to leave Methodist Hospital. This time, I was going home, not to a rehab hospital. I was scared and so was Carole. In a matter of three weeks, I had become accustomed to living at the hospital. In some weird way, Methodist Hospital had become a second home to me, a haven where I felt safe and comfortable. After all, I was being monitored 24/7, including being hooked up to a heart monitor (sort of a security blanket). Going home meant being on my own. So, my paranoia ran rampant. Was I really well enough? What if something happened? Methodist Hospital was an hour's drive away. What if I needed to get back quickly? Would a local hospital do just as well?

Well, it finally came time to wheel me downstairs and to the exit. This time I was in a wheelchair and not being carted around on a gurney. They dropped me off near the patient pickup area, and then Carole and I waited for the valet. It felt strange being outside, almost like this was a brand-new experience. As I sat there, I got nervous, wondering how things would be at home.

After a few minutes, the valet pulled up with Carole's car. I had been told by my doctor that I would have to sit in the back of the car. I would not be able to sit in the front seat for about six weeks, in case the air bags went off (an air bag slamming into my chest would not be good). So, after getting into the car, I began thinking about how fragile my chest must be right now. In response, I kept the shoulder seat belt strap off my chest. I was too scared to allow anything to press against it.

~~~~~~~~~~~~~

The ride home was a bit surreal. I was happy and all, but for some reason, it just didn't feel right. And, even when I got home and saw my house, it felt a bit odd. I couldn't really explain what I was feeling. It was sort of like I was a different person than when I last stepped foot here.

Once inside, I immediately headed to my lounge chair. Besides being anxious, I was still extremely weak and tired. This would become my favorite spot as I recovered, and where I would be for days to come.

As I began to take in everything that had happened to me, I realized that it would take some time for me to adjust to being at home again, as it also would for Carole. That was because Carole, unfortunately, would need to wait on me for the time being. I only hoped she knew how much I appreciated her caring and support.

Sleeping

My first night sleeping at home in my own bed was a blessing, but also a night of fear. Those pesky gerbils in my mind kept running around, creating all sorts of scary thoughts. What if something went wrong? Would I make it through the night? I was not being monitored anymore, so would I know if something started to go wrong? Those thoughts made every twinge, pain, and odd feeling in my chest seem dire. Was that feeling something cardiac related or merely muscular? These thoughts would keep me awake many hours and for plenty of nights to come.

Plus, like in the hospital, I was too scared to sleep on my side for fear of pain or pressure on my aorta and arteries (not that anyone ever told me I couldn't lie on my side, it was just part of my paranoia).
~~~~~~~~~~~~~

So, I forced myself to sleep only on my back, making it hard to get comfortable. And, without the nice pain medications that I got at the hospital, my back hurt. Really hurt. Sleep would not be easy.

Another thing causing me distress in trying to get to sleep was how quiet things were at home. In fact, it was too quiet. At the hospital, there was always some sort of noise to be heard – nurses running around, monitors beeping. So, as I lay there in bed, I could hear my heart pounding. And not just the usual pounding that one normally hears. It was loud. So loud that even Carole could hear it sleeping next to me. But even scarier than hearing my heart pound was feeling it. The intensity of it actually began to shake me. My body rocked in response to the beating of my heart. I wondered if something was wrong, and I began to think that if the beating got any stronger, my heart would burst. But I found out later that this was quite normal after the kind of surgery I had. It would take months before I got comfortable with feeling my heart pounding like this. But, as I heard one person say, "Take comfort in knowing you have a beating heart. It means you're still alive."

The good news was that it was great to be back sleeping with my wife. So, as I lay there, I tried to focus on being home, with Carole, to rid my mind of these nagging fears. She was my rock in all of this.

~~~~~~~~~~~~

Over the next couple of weeks, I would sleep a lot, and I mean a lot, as I became easily fatigued. It would be day and night, and I would sleep as much in my recliner as in my bed. It wasn't that I felt drowsy, it was more that I felt drained, physically exhausted. Carole was surprised at how much I slept. But, as I learned, this too was normal as my body was still healing and recovering from the trauma.

~~~~~~~~~~~~

Eventually, once I got past the initial recovery, I would get to a new normal of sleep mode. I say a new normal because it seems that I won't ever return to my normal sleep pattern that I used to have before my event.

Even though I may sleep in bed for about seven hours, I usually won't actually be asleep any longer than an hour or two at a time. I'll wake up often during the night. I think it's due to my medicines (at least according to one of the side effects), but I'm not sure. Anyway, I've gotten used to it over the past few years.

Feeding Tube

Feeding at home didn't turn out to be as bad as I thought it would be. Having been fed often enough in the hospital, I knew exactly what to do. The hardest part was remembering to open and close the valve (it could be quite messy if you didn't remember). I discovered that it took four full syringes (huge syringes) to inject all of the food from the food supplement carton, and then I injected three full syringes of water (had to stay hydrated). And, in some ways, since I was not hungry for food yet, using the feeding tube was quicker and easier than regular food consumption. Preparation was merely opening up a carton of food, and cleanup was a breeze (as long as I used a cloth in case food leaked out from the syringe).

I felt for Carole, though. Before all of this, we went out to eat a lot. Now, we ate at home. I offered to go out with Carole to a restaurant (I'd eat at home first), but she said that she would feel awkward eating alone. I understood. So, I did the next best thing. When I finally felt strong enough, I cooked dinner for her – meatballs and spaghetti! It was the least I could do after all she had done for me.

There was one place, though, where I did eventually eat out – Methodist Hospital. When I had to go back for tests, it was at times when I had to bring my food with me. Being in the hospital, I didn't feel uneasy feeding myself using the tube. People here should definitely understand. Regardless, though, I still tried to be discreet about it. So, I sat off to the side in the lounge eating area and used the large syringe to feed myself. It made me feel good about myself in that I didn't allow myself to be embarrassed by the ordeal.

~~~~~~~~~~~~~

Wondering what my long-term outlook using a feeding tube was going to be, Carole and I read up on strokes and feeding tubes on the Internet. The prognosis was that this would take a long time before getting back to normal. First, I needed to be approved by a medical professional that I could even attempt to swallow. Then, once I was approved to swallow, I could start swallowing thick liquids (apparently thinner liquids were easier to aspirate). I'd eventually work my way up to swallowing thin liquids. Eating regular food would take more months, again starting with something easy to swallow. It was not a happy thought, but it was something that could be overcome. I kept telling myself how lucky I was to still be alive and that things could be worse (a sentiment that both Carole and I kept repeating to ourselves even to this day). So, I did my best to be grateful. Besides, I was still not hungry for food.

Showering

As in the hospital, I could shower as long as I took some precautions. Before leaving the hospital, Carole and I were told to get a stool for me to sit on in the shower. However, there's a ledge in my shower that I could use if I needed it. Luckily, I was strong enough that I could stand the whole time during my shower, and my balance wasn't "*too*" bad. Nonetheless, I was sure Carole was very nervous for me to be in the shower.

I moved very slowly in the shower (not just because of trying to maintain my balance, but also due to physical pain and being careful not to damage any of my surgical repair). Plus, I had to deal with not getting my feeding tube wet. But, instead of using a large, clear bandage adhered over the feeding tube (as was done in the hospital), Carole helped me put a small towel over the feeding tube and then wrapped me in plastic food wrap (the sticky kind). The wrap wasn't
~~~~~~~~~~~~~

perfect, but it did prove good enough as long as I was careful and did not get myself too soaked. So, until I could get this damn feeding tube out, I dreaded showering. It was a major hassle. After a while, though, I was able to at least start wrapping myself (much to Carole's relief).

Pain

Thankfully, I was still not in too much pain. Which was a very good thing because I was sent home without any pain medications. I was told to take Tylenol as needed, which for the most part did help. I learned that other pain medications, like NSAIDS, could elevate blood pressure so these medications were out of the question (I would learn much about blood pressure in the coming months).

My biggest pain was still my back. Again, my chest only hurt when coughing. I asked my primary care physician for something stronger to help with my back, maybe a muscle relaxer or maybe what they gave me in the hospital for pain – fentanyl. That's when I found out that fentanyl was tightly controlled and was one of the more addictive and deadly drugs being taken illegally. I had heard of it before, but never really knew much about it. Once I learned, I was a bit stunned. Thinking back to when I was given it in the hospital, I remembered how much it helped the pain, but I also remembered how good it made me feel. I understood why people could get addicted to it, and I told myself that it was for the best that my doctor didn't want to prescribe it for me. So, I stuck to Tylenol. I would rather deal with some pain than worry about becoming addicted.

CHAPTER 9: Outpatient Therapy

On September 2nd, exactly one month after my event, I went to Kindred Rehab Hospital for my therapy evaluation. Before starting anything physical, they wanted me to check with my cardiologist about whether I needed cardiac rehab first. Basically, they were worried if I needed medical supervision during my initial rehab to ensure I could handle the exercises. Luckily, my cardiologist said that I didn't need it.

Besides the basic get-back-in-shape need, I told them about my right-hand pain and weakness. In response, they had me do a grip strength test. It showed that my right hand was extremely weak. I also discussed with them about my speech issue and the desire to do another swallow test.

So, for the next few weeks, they signed me up for Physical Therapy, Occupational Therapy, and Speech Therapy.

Physical Therapy

Physical Therapy (PT) was mainly to help me gain strength, stamina, and balance. They started me off with some very basic routines, like slowly walking up and down mini steps, walking on the treadmill, riding a stationary bicycle, and such. For balance, they had me stand on one leg, catch and throw balls, and other activities that would have been childlike if not for the fact that I was having trouble doing them. When I first started, I could see that I needed plenty of improvement. So, I went with the attitude that this was best for me, and I adhered to their instructions.

In addition to the PT, Carole and I began to walk around the neighborhood. It was something Carole had encouraged me to do with her before my event, but something I thought I wouldn't like. Now, it's become one of my favorite things. It's almost like being on a date as we talk about many things. However, as I had learned with everything I now did, something as simple as walking was an ordeal at first.

I found out that besides my muscle weakness and awkwardness, I also had to worry about being dizzy from my vision problems. My dizziness was worse when I looked down, which I tended to do when I walked. So, Carole and I held hands to walk, and not just because we love each other. It was to ensure that I didn't fall down as well as to keep me from veering off the sidewalk (my balance was terrible – I felt like I was in the carnival fun house at times). And don't ask me to look up in the sky or at the moon while walking. I would either end up on the ground or in the neighbor's yard in moments. But, even with all its issues, walking is something that we continue to do to this day (and something I now relish with my wife).

For our first attempt, we only went for a very short walk, just down the block and back. We extended the walks as I became stronger, and now we do a two-mile brisk walk (just under forty minutes) around the neighborhood. An added benefit of walking was that I got to see some of my neighbors, who certainly seemed glad to see me up and about.

[Side note. I discovered that I could not even attempt to jog or run. My balance is so off that I will stumble and fall. I think it is due to my medications. I hope I would never be in a fight-or-flight situation.]

Another issue that my physical therapist helped me with is my vision problem – where I lose focus when trying to look up. First, they directed me to see a neuro-ophthalmologist, Dr. Tang in Houston.

Besides checking out if my eye was causing the problem, she might be able to see if it was something to do with my brain (maybe from my two strokes?). Second, they gave me a list of eye exercises that I could do that might help me adapt. These exercises involved looking side to side, up-down, down-up, diagonally to diagonally. Only the down-up gave me an issue, which I found strange.

Occupational Therapy

Occupational Therapy was to mainly work with the use of my right hand. Besides some exercises to strengthen my hand, they had me undergo sensory applications to try to help alleviate the pain (besides the intense pain when I rubbed my hand, there was a constant dull ache – this aching was also part of the problem with trying to get to sleep). One sensory application was to stick my hand in some warm sawdust-like material. The feeling was very soothing. Another activity was for me to use my right hand to try to pick up certain small objects one at a time. I had a lot of difficulty with this as it was hard for me to squeeze my thumb and forefinger together. In fact, I couldn't even make a fist. They also gave me a squeeze ball to work with at home. To help with my pain, they gave me a compression glove to wear at home. Surprisingly, it did provide some relief, at least enough to help me get to sleep at night.

Speech Therapy

Speech Therapy was to mainly help me with exercising my tongue and throat muscles so that I could eventually swallow. But I was also self-conscious about the way I sounded when I spoke. Words seemed to linger on my tongue as I tried to say them, and certain sounds needed to be retrained altogether. Plus, since I couldn't get the words out sometimes, I'd stutter.

To accomplish that, my speech therapist coached me on trying to speak and utter various sounds. Apparently, the tongue has a major influence on swallowing. So, to activate and strengthen my tongue and throat muscles, I had to recite certain words and create all sorts of weird noises. I learned which words worked on the tip of the tongue, the middle of the tongue, and the back of the tongue. I was also given various tongue exercises, like sticking your tongue out in certain directions or trying to curl the tip of your tongue up and down (something I found very hard to do). I also discovered that when I stuck out my tongue, it curved to the side instead of staying straight. I learned later that this was a typical sign of having had a stroke. Through it all, I learned a lot about speech in general. I found it all very interesting.

The recitation of the sounds and words required a lot of repetition. Do twenty of that. Do thirty of those. I even had to do tongue twisters, like "Sally sells seashells…" To hear me utter some of these sounds was quite amusing. Instead of being embarrassed, though, I ended up laughing at myself. Again, I wanted to do what was necessary to reach my goal. Plus, I tried very hard not to criticize my current disability.

One other technique used was something called a Transcutaneous Electrical Nerve Stimulation (TENS) unit. It was a small electrode that attached to the base of my throat, and it emitted electrical impulses to stimulate the nerves and muscles. The intensity started off low and could be ramped up. To get the best result, I needed to have it near the max. When I first tried it, it felt weird, a strange tingling sensation. By the time I got near the max intensity, it began to hurt. It even burned a little. My therapist said that I wasn't getting a smooth enough contact between the device and my skin due to my beard growth. She suggested that I try to shave more closely before wearing it the next time. However, it still burned even with a closer shave. I tried to endure it in the hopes it was helping. Then, one day, I experienced A-fib. I didn't know what caused the A-fib, but it happened after I started using the TENS unit. I told my speech therapist that I thought it might be the device. She didn't think so, but being paranoid, I stopped using it anyway.

Good to Eat

As in my final days at Methodist Hospital, I kept asking to have another swallowing test. It had been several days since my earlier test, and even though I was not supposed to, I had been trying very small sips of water at home and hadn't gagged once. (Yay!) I didn't tell Kindred Hospital that, but I pushed to have another test, eager to see if I was really getting better. However, Kindred Hospital needed to have a doctor present, and it took a few days before one could be scheduled.

On September 14th, almost two weeks into rehab, I finally got my wish. One of their doctors had time to oversee my swallow test. So, an alternate speech therapist pulled me into an x-ray room. When the doctor arrived, I was given a liquid to swallow while he x-rayed my throat. Not sure what to expect, I was a little nervous. But thank God I didn't have any trouble swallowing. The doctor told me that everything appeared normal, and the speech therapist informed me that I could start eating. After reading about stroke victims online, Carole asked, "What can he eat?" Both she and I assumed that I would need to start out with some type of liquid diet. To our surprise, the speech therapist said that I can eat anything I wanted to, that the imaging showed my throat muscles were working normally. Apparently, my swallowing trouble was due to muscle atrophy all along, and not from my strokes. Carole and I were ecstatic. This was great news.

So, to celebrate that I could finally eat, later that same day, Carole and I went to one of my favorite Mexican restaurants, Mr. Sombrero's, and I ordered Enchiladas Verde. I was still hesitant, so I started off very slow and careful. But, as I was told earlier, I could swallow. I savored every bite. Aahhhh! I also enjoyed every swallow of water. What a blessing! It really made me think about not taking everyday capabilities for granted. I mean, who really thinks that you might lose the ability to drink and eat? It's not until you lose something that's so basic before you understand true gratitude. Maybe this was a lesson that God wanted me to learn.

Mouth Control

However, even though I could now eat, I kept going to the speech therapist. I still needed to work on my speech. Plus, there were some related problems to deal with, ones involving mouth strength and control.

The first problem was drooling. Sometimes when I leaned over, I couldn't contain the drool in my mouth, and it leaked out. That's a little embarrassing.

The second problem (which wasn't anything detrimental) was that I couldn't whistle. Even now, years later, after regaining most of my mouth control, I still find it very difficult to whistle.

The third problem was the worst. Now that I was eating again, I discovered that my bite was sometimes off, or rather I had episodes of uncontrollable muscle contractions, causing my mouth to involuntarily bite down. It became quite apparent that my lack of tongue control also affected my mouth control, including how I chewed. I would randomly bite the side of my cheek, my lip, my tongue, and even my front teeth (it was so bad once that I actually chipped one of my front teeth, which required it to be glued back on). The most painful was biting my tongue. I cringed in pain each time that happened. Once, I almost bit off a small chunk of my tongue. It bled pretty well. Luckily, your mouth heals quickly. Unfortunately, this happened so often that I usually had a sore somewhere on the inside of my mouth.

So, getting better tongue control was really needed, and my speech therapist gave me plenty of tongue and mouth exercises (like using a straw to suck and hold a cotton ball). However, the best exercise for getting better at eating was to eat. I just needed to try to be careful. But, even when I concentrated on chewing, I could still bite wrong. My muscles would twitch or spasm or something. I read online that there are neurological disorders that could cause this. Whatever it was, it was something that I didn't appear to have control over, and sometimes I don't think I ever will. Because, even to this day, I still occasionally bite wrong.

PEG Tube Out

Also, now that I could finally eat, I scheduled an appointment with Dr. Schwarz, my gastroenterologist, to see about getting my PEG tube taken out. I didn't use it for feeding anymore, and it was a pain to have, especially when showering.

On September 26th, I went in to see Dr. Schwarz. I was scared about getting the tube pulled. How much would it hurt? Would I have a hole that needed to be sutured? Would I have to wait to eat again for it to heal?

So, when Dr. Schwarz came in and had me lie on the table to examine me, I tried to relax. I felt him checking the tube as he nonchalantly talked to Carole and me. Then, all of a sudden, he said it was done. Confused, I asked, "What's done?" He said that he had already pulled out my PEG tube. I couldn't believe it. I didn't feel a thing. He then put a bandage over the hole and informed me to keep the bandage on for a day or so. I asked if I could eat. He said of course, but I shouldn't overeat for a couple of days. He said that there shouldn't be any leakage. I was amazed. And overjoyed. My PEG tube was out! One more step closer to being normal.

Driving

With my recovery going well, one of my next concerns was about driving. I knew that even riding in a car was dangerous for me until about six weeks, but with my dizziness when walking and my vision coordination problem, I was scared if I would ever be able to drive again. If, for some reason, I couldn't drive, then would I be able to return to work? Plus, because of my condition, this meant that Carole had to drive all the time. Not that she had a problem driving, but normally I was the one that drove us around. So, for several weeks, Carole was my chauffeur. Not a role she was particularly fond of. This included driving me back and forth to Methodist Hospital in Houston, in horrendous highway traffic. Again, God gave her the strength she needed.

I asked one of the trainers at Kindred if they provided therapy to help get me back to driving. I was told that they didn't. They recommended that when I thought I was ready, that I should just go with someone to a parking lot and give it a try.

So, while waiting a few weeks to regain my strength and confidence, I took much more interest in how I saw out of the car while riding with Carole. I noticed that I had no problem looking straight ahead or looking to the sides. But, due to my vision problem, my issue was only when I looked down and then back up. It took me a moment before getting things in focus. This meant that I would have issues trying to read the speedometer or any other vehicle data and then try to look back up at the road again.

Carole and I discussed my options. As far as work went, I could either check to see if my employer would accommodate me working from home, or I would have to see if I could drive. But driving was more than just about getting to work. It was freedom, and it alleviated Carole from having to be my personal chauffeur.

So, after my six weeks to heal, and when I finally felt ready, I went for a test drive – just a short drive from my house to our community clubhouse, maybe a half mile away. I was a little nervous, but also eager. I tried not to think about it too much. When I began to back out of our garage, I immediately discovered that my feel of the car was off (I attributed this to my balance being off). Because of this, I turned the car too soon. The front of the car clipped a cabinet along the side of our garage. I was going slow enough that I didn't damage the car, but the one side of the cabinet was almost torn off. With things starting badly, I was worried if I could really do this, but I knew that I needed to keep going. I regained my focus and backed out onto the street. I then drove the short distance to the clubhouse. While driving, I tried looking down at the speedometer and then back up. It took me a moment to readjust my vision, but I was able to see quickly enough that I didn't think this would be an issue. No other issues were encountered. I considered this a good first trial.

With the test drive successful, I attempted further driving around town, just short drives. But it wasn't long before I got comfortable with driving, including my vision problem. And it wasn't long before I began driving on my own. However, the first time that I needed to drive on the highway, I got a bit nervous. Luckily, things went well. As time went on, I would get accustomed to my vision problem to the point that I didn't even think about it anymore. I still have the problem, but I have endured it for so long that I automatically adjust my eyes to it. It's amazing how your body (and mind) adapts.

CHAPTER 10: More Complications

Heart Palpitations

One day, not too long after being able to eat, on the way to breakfast, I began to experience constant heart palpitations. That's that fluttering feeling in your chest like your heart is skipping a beat or beginning to go haywire. It's bad enough when you get a single skip. I've had those before. But this time, the palpitations kept coming. It was scary.

I told Carole about it and mentioned that it had been going on for at least fifteen minutes. We didn't know if this was something serious or not. We were almost to our destination, but then I began thinking that maybe we should head home in case I needed to go to the ER.

On the way back, instead of going home, we drove to the local hospital instead. I was still debating how bad my palpitations were. We pulled into the hospital's parking lot and sat there discussing whether I should go in and get checked out. I was really afraid, but was what I was feeling really an emergency? As we talked, I finally realized that I had not taken my morning medications yet (I was too eager to get to breakfast). I checked my heart rate and it seemed okay, so at least we didn't think I was going into A-fib. We eventually decided to go home, take my medicines, and see what would happen. If the medicines didn't help, or if things got worse, I could still always go to the hospital.

Well, not long after taking my medicines, the palpitations finally went away. What a relief, and what a lesson to learn.

~~~~~~~~~~~~~

We found out later that heart palpitations are common after major heart surgery and severe trauma to the heart. However, my cardiologist, to be sure it wasn't A-fib, put me on a heart monitor for a month.

Wearing the heart monitor wasn't so bad, at least with this one, since it was not hardwired. The small monitor merely stuck on your chest and used radio waves to communicate with a tracking device – a smartphone that talked with the monitoring company.

As luck (or not) would have it, no further heart palpitations occurred while I was on the heart monitor. So, this was chalked up to a one-time experience.

Heartburn & Racing Heart

After a few weeks at home, I began to experience heartburn. I didn't expect to have heartburn because I was already on a Proton Pump Inhibitor (PPI) – forty mg Pantoprazole twice a day, due to Barrett's esophagus. Well, I started taking some chewable antacids. Over the next few days, the heartburn continued, and I continued taking more antacids. I didn't understand why this was happening.

Then, one day, driving home from the pharmacy, my heart suddenly began to race, and not just beat a little bit faster. It beat so fast that I thought I might pass out. I became extremely scared. Only minutes away from home, I worried if I would be able to make it. I wondered if I should pull off the road and call 911. Luckily, my heart stopped racing within several seconds. Of course, it felt much longer.
~~~~~~~~~~~~~

Carole and I debated whether I should contact my cardiologist. As with the palpitations, was this a one-time thing? So, we decided to wait and see if it would happen again.

Well, it did. One morning, as I was about to eat breakfast, my heart began to race again. It felt like it did the last time, and my fear instantly rose. Being at home, I quickly checked my blood pressure and heart rate. My heart rate had jumped to 150 bpm (normally it is in the sixties or seventies). Not good.

This time, I contacted my cardiologist. He had me wear that heart monitor again to check for A-fib. And, as before, I did not have any more episodes while on the monitor. A part of me was actually disappointed since I was looking for answers, but another part was quite happy that it didn't happen again.

~~~~~~~~~~~~~

In the meantime, Carole and I looked on the Internet and found several possible reasons for my racing heart. One bit of information we came across was that one of my medicines, Metoprolol, could affect the Lower Esophageal Sphincter (LES) muscle, making it weaker. This could be the cause of my indigestion and heartburn. Another item we came across was that calcium could interfere with Metoprolol. Hmmmm! The antacids I was taking were basically calcium. With the amount of antacids I took, I deduced that I was negating the effects of my Metoprolol. So, I stopped taking the antacids. In response, I didn't experience any more racing heart. That was the good news. The bad news was that I still had heartburn. So, I made an appointment with my gastroenterologist, Dr. Schwarz.

~~~~~~~~~~~~~

I told Dr. Schwarz about my problem, and that I thought it was the Metoprolol causing my heartburn. First, he wanted to do another endoscopy to make sure there was no new damage from all of my heartburn. He also prescribed me a second stomach medicine – 150 mg Ranitidine twice a day.

Well, the endoscopy showed everything was okay (great!), and after starting the Ranitidine, my heartburn went away.

Just another instance where one medicine led to additional troubles and additional medicines. I swear that half of my medicines are to resolve issues caused by the other half of my medicines.

Vision Problem & TIAs

In response to my vision focus problems, I made an appointment with Dr. Tang, a neuro-ophthalmologist.

Right before my appointment, I experienced something weird. Coming home from the store, as I carried in a case of water, a gray spot appeared in my right eye. It partially blinded me in that I could not see through the gray spot (I could see all around it, though). I could not rub it away, and nothing I did seemed to affect it.

I started thinking that maybe this was due to carrying in the water. Was the water too heavy for me to carry? The case of water must have weighed about forty pounds. I got very worried. Maybe I exerted myself too much and my blood pressure spiked. I immediately went and took my blood pressure. Thankfully, it was okay. Regardless, I sat down and rested.

After about five or ten minutes, the gray spot disappeared, and my right eye was fine. Without any other symptoms, I didn't think much about it. I did try to look up what it could be on the Internet. Barring other symptoms, it was hard to tell what it might have been. I was thinking (or really hoping) that it might have been some type of ocular migraine or such. Some of the other choices on the Internet weren't so good.

~~~~~~~~~~~~~
~~~~~~~~~~~~~

In that same week, I visited Dr. Tang hoping to learn what might have been causing my vision problem. I told her about what was going on, but I also mentioned to her about the gray spot in my right eye (again, I wasn't thinking that it was anything critical). First, she did plenty of tests, some of which I had never seen before. But second, she was concerned that my right eye episode was due to a Transient Ischemic Attack (TIA). A TIA could interrupt blood flow to the eye, which would explain my gray spot. She said that if it was a TIA then it could be a precursor to a stroke. She wanted me to go to the hospital immediately after leaving her office to get it checked out. Carole and I were skeptical, still thinking that I would have had other symptoms if it were a TIA, like speech problems or confusion or something. To aid in her concern, Dr. Tang called my cardiologist, Dr. Zoghbi, who apparently was also concerned. Both doctors wanted me to go to the hospital – ASAP. So, even though I wasn't really convinced, Carole and I headed over to Methodist Hospital once done with Dr. Tang.

After checking in at the Methodist Hospital ER, Carole and I headed to the waiting room, and waited. And waited. And waited. After at least an hour, Carole and I decided that since I didn't have any other symptoms for the last few days, this was a waste of time. I checked out and we headed home.

In response to this episode, Dr. Zoghbi called me afterward and put me on full-dose aspirin as a precaution. I was fine with that.

~~~~~~~~~~~~~

I would experience one more episode of a gray spot in my right eye, and like before, it only lasted for a few minutes. And, without any other symptoms, I still didn't seek help. My stubbornness and arrogance ruled. I just wasn't sure what the hospital could do other than monitor me.

~~~~~~~~~~~~~

What I learned much later is that Dr. Tang was probably correct in that what I experienced were TIAs, and I shouldn't have taken them so casually. Luckily, I didn't experience any more of these episodes and I haven't noticed any ill effects from them. Things could have definitely been worse if these TIAs were a precursor to a stroke. But, fortunately for me, they weren't. My luck was still with me. But how long could I rely on luck?

From what I gathered, there were several possible causes for these TIAs after my dissection event; the most probable was contamination from the heart/lung bypass machine (at least in my opinion).

CHAPTER 11: Return to Work

While I was in the hospital, Carole was the one who dealt with my employer, The Boeing Company. Luckily, she was friends with one of my coworkers, so she had called her to inform Boeing of what happened to me. That led to Carole dealing with Boeing's Human Resources (HR) personnel. Part of what Carole had to do was get paperwork filled out by Methodist Hospital to put me on medical leave. And, after using up all of my sick time, I needed to go on short-term disability, which meant more paperwork.

[*I really admire Carole for taking this on because she hates doing this type of thing (actually, so do I).*]

Well, it turned out that Carole had to communicate with Boeing a lot, at least until I got home. Then, I was able to deal with Boeing.

~~~~~~~~~~~~~

It would take me three and a half months before I finally felt strong enough to return to work. After being off for so long, and with depression settling in from my event, I really didn't want to return. But there was no easy way for me to live on what Carole and I had saved so far.

So, to ease my way back, I talked with Boeing to see if I might start out with a reduced schedule – work half days for a couple of weeks, then three-quarter days, and finally full time by the end of December
~~~~~~~~~~~~~

(just in time to take off about two weeks for the holiday break). They were fine with that as long as I had a doctor's recommendation. So, I contacted my cardiologist, Dr. Zoghbi, and he was good with my request. I have to say that Boeing is a great employer to allow me such flexibility. They have great benefits.

As I expected, it was an adjustment going back to work. I was a software engineer working for Boeing on the International Space Station Project. And even though my job allowed me to sit at a desk, I found that I still got easily fatigued. It would take time for me to build up my endurance. But I knew that I was extremely lucky that I could still work. I didn't think about it, but Carole was worried that with my two strokes, would I be able to perform my job well enough? Would I still have the same cognitive abilities? It didn't take me long to see that I could still perform my job. Another gratitude to thank God.

My only difficulty I encountered in returning to work was the need to control my anxiety and blood pressure (like confrontations at meetings). As already mentioned, I had been noticing a slight change in personality (PTSD or stroke or both?), and I had become somewhat intolerant of others. It took much effort to overcome this shortfall, but after a time, I adjusted. Part of my adjustment was to leave a situation if things ever got too intense. I told myself that trying to influence work situations just wasn't worth my life.

One interesting thing was that, previously, I was manager over my software team. Due to company downsizing, I was forced to change positions (this was all prior to my event). At the time, I was very bitter about the move, thinking how unfair it was. After all, in some ways, it was truly a demotion. But, as Carole and I discussed after my event, that demotion was a blessing in disguise. I didn't think I could have handled all the stress of being a manager and kept my blood pressure down. I like to think now that God was preparing me for my future. This would be the beginning of more realizations about God's influence over me as time goes on.

CHAPTER 12: My New Normal

My "new normal." When I first heard the term, I didn't really understand it. I didn't realize that my life was about to change drastically. Some for the worse, but some was actually for the better. Of course, as with everything in life, it was one's perspective of things that really matters. The problem was trying to work past all of the new setbacks and focus on all that was good in my life.

What was funny was Carole and I didn't realize the extent of my damage until after a further detailed reading of my test results. Initially, I was so ecstatic to have survived, and I had thought I was fixed. I mean, isn't that what surgery usually does – fix you? It wasn't that I thought that I was back to normal (at least not yet), but I thought that after I healed completely, I would be fine – back to how I was before. But that was before understanding what really happened to me. I knew that I had an aneurysm that ruptured, and something was said about being dissected. But I didn't realize that my aorta was still dissected and would stay that way – FOREVER! I guess I thought that my aorta would heal like any other wound. That isn't the case with a dissection.

There was plenty to read from my test results. Things like a false lumen. So, Carole and I began to research all of this on the Internet, which wasn't always a good thing. But we did learn much about the terminology contained in my test results. However, with that knowledge, more questions arose. Mainly, what was my prognosis?

How long could I expect to live? The Internet cited studies that weren't very promising. Things like high morbidity rate in the first year or two, and life expectancy beyond ten years didn't seem likely.

Well, this caused Carole and me a lot of anxiety and depression. The doctors had seemed very pleased with my response so far, but now I began to think that maybe my survival was fleeting. So much so, that I didn't even think it wise to buy a calendar for the next year. After all, why waste money on something that I might not be able to fully use? I also didn't want to buy personal items as well. Things like new clothes. What was the use? I then started thinking that maybe I might have enough time to at least get my affairs in order. Like what personal stuff of mine I should I throw out so Carole wouldn't have to fool with it when I died? Carole must have had similar thoughts too, because after having to pay the bills and handle other matters while I was in the hospital, she wanted to know all I did. This wasn't a great way to live – to constantly worry that you might die in the very near future.

This wasn't the only change in my life. As already stated, even though my aortic valve and ascending aorta had been fixed, I still lived with a dissection to the rest of my aorta down into my right iliac artery. Because of this, I had to make lifestyle changes to always keep my blood pressure and heart rate under control. Because of my weakened aortic walls, new aneurysms could develop. So, in addition to my cardiac surgeon, I also had to continue seeing my cardiologist. Dr. Zoghbi. I would have to visit both of these doctors on a regular basis, for the rest of my life, to check my aorta. There is the very real possibility that I might need more surgery in the future.

So, besides worrying about whether I would die soon, I also worried if I would get another aneurysm or dissection, or if my graft would even last. The only good news in all of this was that, unlike the vast majority of people, I would now be having my aorta monitored so that, hopefully, I would know beforehand if another aneurysm began to grow. Lucky me.

Blood Pressure (BP)

Because of the threat of having another aneurysm, I became very self-conscious about my blood pressure and heart rate, including limiting how much weight I lifted, how much exercising I did, and how much stress I allowed. Of course, stress wasn't something that you could easily avoid in life. I knew that this was something I would have to live with for the rest of my life.

So, I constantly checked my blood pressure, almost to the point of being obsessive. At first, I started checking it daily, even multiple times a day, scared that whatever I was doing might be causing my BP to rise. The goal was to keep my BP at 120/70 or even lower, and to not allow my systolic to get above 140. To help accomplish this, my cardiologist had me on multiple blood pressure medicines.

When I left the hospital, I was on ten mg Amlodipine (a calcium channel blocker) for blood pressure, and 300 mg Metoprolol Tartrate (a beta-blocker) for blood pressure, heart rate, and heart arrhythmias. Over the past few years, the Metoprolol was reduced to 200 mg, and I have added 2.5 mg Lisinopril (mainly for my kidneys, but it also helps with blood pressure) and eight mg Cardura for blood pressure. Surprisingly, all of these BP meds did not make me tired.

[*Because of all my medical conditions, I have a drawer full of medications and supplements; all but a couple have been prescribed by a doctor. To date, I have thirteen prescriptions and ten supplements I take every day.*]

However, these medicines could only do so much. A lot depended not only on my physical activities, but also on my emotional state as well. Needless to say, getting angry or uptight was not healthy. It could be lethal. So, every time something or someone pissed me off, I had to tell myself that it wasn't worth risking my life over (which is easier said than done when some jerk cuts you off in traffic). I also concluded that I was much calmer when I didn't watch the news (not really surprising).

I also had to be very careful about using any medications, eating certain foods, and drinking any beverages that might raise my blood pressure or interact with my current medications. Caffeine, for sure, was on my DO NOT USE list. But so were medicines like pseudoephedrine and NSAIDs. For the most part, this wasn't bad, but there were times (like when I got a really bad sinus headache) when I really wished things were different. Because of my restrictions, Tylenol became my new best friend. That, or tough out the pain.

Physical Limitations & Exercise

Originally, when I first came home, I was told by my cardiac surgeon that I could not lift anything over twenty pounds. Twenty pounds? That wasn't very much weight. Until I thought about it, there was a lot I couldn't do anymore with a restriction like that (suitcases, laundry baskets, grocery bags, etc.). I felt like an invalid, but considering the risk, I adhered to the restriction as best I could. Of course, when I first got home, it wasn't too hard to follow since I slept a lot. Unfortunately, poor Carole had to do most of the work around the house.

Later, after finishing my rehab, my cardiologist told me that I could exercise, but only if I use light weights (no more than seven pounds), and also if I did not strain myself. In fact, I should never strain myself doing anything, including going to the bathroom. Can you imagine dying in the bathroom? That's not how I wanted to die. One of the best things I could do, though, was walking, but I had to keep my heart rate below 110 bpm.

So, I started exercising at a very slow pace – ten minutes of walking at two miles/hour, a few very light resistant machines, and only five-pound weights. I tracked my BP and heart rate excessively to make sure I was doing okay. And it appeared that everything was fine. I gradually increased my regimen to thirty minutes of brisk walking (3.6 miles/hour) and twenty minutes of light resistance machines using weights no heavier than eight pounds. It wasn't close to what

I used to do, but I was comfortable with this. One interesting thing that I noticed was how doing aerobic exercise temporarily lowered my BP. For me, it was around twenty to thirty points lower.

Once I felt like I'd gained some strength (several weeks later), I started doing minimal housework and yard work. It was just the very basics, but even that was tiring. I easily become exhausted. It was amazing to see how out of shape I had become. It took time, but I was able to do more and more as the weeks went by. But, to keep my blood pressure low, I purposely took my time and took plenty of rests.

Eventually, I asked my cardiologist if it was okay to lift something heavier, like a suitcase (you wouldn't believe how much things weigh until you have restrictions). He said that an occasional one-time lift (as in loading a fifty-pound suitcase into the car trunk) was okay as long as I wasn't straining myself. This gave me some leeway, but initially I was still very self-conscious each time I lifted anything remotely heavy. Over time, though, as I did more and more, I found it easy to start becoming complacent. I had to keep reminding myself of my limitations. Which is not that simple when you feel physically able to do something, and the only thing keeping you from not doing anything too strenuous is your memory. Because most of the time, you don't feel high blood pressure.

Chest Pains & Discomforts

Heart palpitations were not the only scary feelings I had. I experienced many weird and scary chest feelings, discomforts, and pain. Most were likely due to the major surgery of having my chest cracked open and wired shut. I was able to convince myself that some of the odd feelings had to be muscular, since I had no other heart-related symptoms (like shortness of breath or dizziness).

Other odd feelings I would also dismiss since I didn't experience any issues while exercising (my rudimentary thinking was that if I had cardiac issues, they should show up under physical stress). Even so,

I came very close to going to the ER a few times, scared that something serious was happening. And for anyone thinking that my logic was medically good to use, please don't. Just because I had fared okay so far, didn't mean that what I did was correct, as will be seen later. Anyone wondering if what is going on with them might be bad, especially with known medical issues, please go to the ER. As someone else said, "The ER doctor would rather see you twenty times for nothing than once to pronounce you dead."

Pump Head

Another new term – Pump Head. It refers to the cognitive decline caused by being hooked up to the heart/lung bypass machine. For me, it meant that my memory wasn't what it used to be. I found myself forgetting things much more often, mainly short-term memory. Carole would start talking about a conversation we had, and I'd look at her like "What?" Thankfully, she knew that my memory problems were not my fault. Not that it wasn't frustrating for her, but at least she knew that I wasn't ignoring her.

Cold

I noticed that I was feeling cold all the time. I knew that I was slightly anemic due to my kidney disease, but this feeling of cold was worse. I read that some people who had been on the heart/lung bypass machine experience problems with their body temperatures, or at least what their temperature feels like. I also read others had complained about the temperature side effects of beta-blockers. Regardless of why, I felt cold. A lot. I constantly used a throw blanket on me while watching television, and I pulled up the comforter at night when in bed. I also felt much more comfortable if I wore a light jacket even when the temperature outside wasn't that cool. This also included many restaurants and grocery stores as well (don't know why they keep their establishments so cold).

Then, there was the time Carole and I went to a neighbor's party out on their deck. It was winter, but being in Texas, it wasn't really that cold outside. However, after staying outside for a short while, I eventually had to go inside. And stay inside. I was shivering so hard my chest began to hurt. I could not stand the cold, even with my winter coat on.

Carole and I would laugh about all of this, but part of me felt like the stereotypical elderly person wearing their sweater in the middle of summer. It made me feel self-conscious. So, at times when we'd go walking in our neighborhood, I would tell Carole, "Don't worry. I won't embarrass you by wearing my jacket." Even though I may have wished I had.

Alcohol

After a while, I wondered how I would react if I had an alcoholic drink. Now that I could eat again and go out to a restaurant, having a drink would be nice. Plus, like many people, Carole didn't wish to drink alone. I was worried, though, about how alcohol would react with my new medicines, especially the blood pressure ones. I had read online that alcohol could amplify the effects of these medicines. So, before going out for a drink, I decided to try a drink at home, in case things didn't go too well. After all, I wouldn't want Carole having to call 911 at the restaurant because I passed out due to too low of a BP. So, I opened up a bottle of wine and poured Carole and myself a glass. Luckily for me, I didn't notice anything different than when I used to drink before. I was happy. As long as I kept my drinking to a moderate level, I was fine.

Intimacy

One other scary first was sex. I wanted to give it a try even though I wasn't sure about it being safe. After all, I was a normal male. But Carole was way too scared, to the point that she wouldn't even entertain the idea of sex until my doctor gave me permission. I understood. Besides the trauma of another event happening, I was sure Carole didn't want to explain to the EMTs how it happened.

So, when it came time for my first follow-up in September, I asked my cardiac surgeon, Dr. Reardon, if it was okay for me to be intimate with my wife. He quipped that as long as I wasn't tossing Carole around, I would be okay. He said that as long as the sex wasn't strenuous, there shouldn't be any reason that I couldn't.

Well, I was ecstatic. Carole was still scared, though. So, when the time came that we finally were intimate, we were very careful, and took things slowly. Immediately afterward, I checked my blood pressure. My BP was reasonable, and I didn't experience any issues.

As time went on, and our love life resumed, nothing out of the ordinary occurred. Carole eventually became comfortable with the idea that I would be fine.

However, there was one problem, though – Erectile Dysfunction (ED). Being on multiple heart medications is hell on ED. As such, there wasn't much hope in keeping things normal, at least until my body got used to my medications. It took a while, but improvisation, patience, and acceptance of one's limitations were key to having a good sex life. The hardest part was trying not to think about my *problem* during sex. Pressure to finish in time before things went bad only worsened the issue. (I think the mental aspect became a bigger issue than the physical.) Over time, though, I relented to the fact that things would not work out every time. Once I came to terms with that, I felt much better. My biggest fear was that my wife would think less of me. But she was still grateful that I was even around. I am so lucky to have an understanding wife.

Other People

Another thing that bothered me (but, at times, gave me some amusing satisfaction) was talking to others about my condition. What was funny was that no matter what I said, most people thought I had had a heart attack, or at least equated it to something similar to a heart attack. That's because most people had never heard of an aortic dissection, and therefore they don't understand how different the two conditions are. I couldn't blame them since I never knew about it before either.

But because some people thought that my dissection was similar to other types of heart disease, I would get asked about my restrictions, especially concerning my diet. This happened a lot if I ate anything remotely bad. I'd hear, "You can eat that?"

Another annoying thing was that people did not understand that I would never be completely healed. Of course, I didn't realize that at first either, but even when I told people I was still dissected, they dismissed it since I appeared normal. I guess I should have been thankful that I was well enough that I didn't exhibit any infirmity. The issue with this was that people just didn't understand that I couldn't do everything I used to do, particularly with physical activity.

Plus, many people, when they asked, "How are you doing?" usually meant physically. They didn't really want to know how I was doing emotionally, which was most of my problem. So, I usually told people, "I'm doing fine, *considering*." I did not go into what "considering" meant. So far, no one has ever asked me to explain.

Holidays

When the holidays came (just weeks after my surgery), they were severely muted. It was hard enough that I had physical limitations, but the emotional drain was terrible. Remember, I was still in the mindset of wondering if I would survive another year. Trying to get into the holiday spirit was not possible. Carole and I put up only a very few decorations. Which, if you know me, was completely uncharacteristic. Carole was likewise depressed, and I was just trying to cope through it all.

Things would get better in the following years, thank God. So, by the third Christmas after my event, things were almost back to normal, including actually enjoying the holidays and putting up many more decorations. The only real difference was our Christmas tree. With my physical restriction, having a seven-foot tree was not a good idea anymore. So, we got rid of our large artificial tree and bought a much smaller one, a four-foot tree. Carole liked it better anyway since there was less to decorate on the tree.

Travel

Another phobia I developed was to travel, at least to any place that was even the slightest bit remote. I now feared being too far from a major hospital, just in case another emergency happened. It didn't matter how good I felt, or how healthy I thought I was. And, for the very near future, taking any trip overseas was definitely out of the question. I kept thinking about how things might be if something similar happened while on a cruise, or in another country. So, for the near term, I would only consider domestic travel to cities with a renowned hospital.

~~~~~~~~~~~~~

For my first Christmas after my event, Carole and I considered going to New York City. We had already booked reservations prior to my event. I was nervous, as I already said, but I knew Carole was eager to go, and we both needed a break. So, after my follow-up MRA in September, I asked my cardiac surgeon, Dr. Reardon, if it was okay for me to fly. He quipped that it was okay as long as I wasn't the one flying the plane.

Well, Carole and I flew to NYC, even though I was nervous the whole time. The plane ride itself was scary. Without any valid reason, I feared that the cabin pressure change might somehow do something to my dissected aorta. Of course, that didn't happen, but fears are fears. They are real to you at the time. Plus, I also feared the development of a blood clot, thereby causing a stroke. That didn't happen either. Damn mind gerbils.

When we arrived in NYC, we took a cab to our hotel, the New York Marriott Marquis in the heart of Times Square. When we got near to the hotel, the traffic was horrendous. I kept thinking, what if I needed to get to the hospital? An ambulance would never make it in
~~~~~~~~~~~~~

time. Could they do life flight? I tried my best to push that thought aside.

To add to my distress, a cold front came through, bringing a very wet snow. Sensitive to the cold, I was freezing. All in all, though, I managed to enjoy our stay. That didn't mean that I still didn't dread the plane ride home. Who needed carnival rides for a thrill when you have a serious medical condition?

~~~~~~~~~~~~~

Besides traveling, my phobia of being too far from a hospital also got me thinking of people who live remotely, out in the boonies, or even in a small city. I wondered what happens to them if something similar occurs. There were times in the past that I used to daydream of living remotely in some beautiful, fantasy landscape. No more.

PTSD & Depression

Well, as might be evident, my emotional health seemed to be worse than my physical health. With the constant worry of controlling my blood pressure, limiting my physical activities, getting freaked out with every chest discomfort, and thinking that I could die at any time, it wasn't a surprise that I went into a depression. I realized that I also probably had PTSD from my near-death experience, and all of this was overshadowing everything in my life.

But, besides the turmoil of my inner emotional state, I began to exhibit external traits too. I became jealous of others who were in good health and could do whatever they wanted. This led me to start becoming intolerant of others. It irritated me when I heard others complain about trivial things in their lives. And, since I felt like I had just been cheated in life, a sourness rose in me.

Many of my dreams and daydreams were gone, knowing that I could never be too physical again. Contact sports were out of the question. Body building was a no-no. And any fantasy that involved being too active was now no longer enjoyable. After all, part of a good fantasy
~~~~~~~~~~~~~

was thinking that it was somehow possible, no matter how unlikely. Now, if one of these fantasies came to mind, my first thought was "That's stupid; I'd most likely die doing that." I knew that some of these daydreams (and bucket list items) were silly ones, ones that I'd never do, but just knowing that they were now impossible made me feel like I had lost a part of my life.

This sourness affected me to the point that if anyone wronged me (at least in my mind), no matter how small, I became irate. I already lost enough and what little else remained, even if just fantasies, had somehow become critical. Carole saw my changed behavior and told me about it. She was worried. I tried working on being more like my old self, but it was hard. At least I was now aware of it.

Another aspect of my PTSD was that I had become very sensitive. I would start crying at the drop of a hat. And, it didn't have to be due to some intense, emotional event. And it didn't matter if it was good or bad. Just a simple emotional provocation and the tears began. I'd get a birthday card, and I'd start thinking how lucky I was to be alive. Next thing I knew, tears were running down my face. The slightest touching moment on a TV show and I struggled not to cry. I used to be a sensitive person before, but nothing like this. Now, I had a hard time controlling my emotions. Even to this day, though not as often, I will still cry whenever I encounter something emotional.

I need to also point out that Carole was also experiencing her own PTSD. Like me, she had become very concerned about my health and was deathly afraid that I might die at any moment. Considering that there was no warning sign of my dissection/aneurysm, just because I seemed fine at the moment meant nothing (a small part of me also thought that I could die at any moment). Only with time did the constant worry (for her and me) begin to ease. I tried to put myself in her shoes to think what I would have been like, and I was amazed at her strength. Like she told me, we are all stronger than we think when put to the test.

But because I understood her worry, I did what I could to ease her mind. That included things like letting her know that I had arrived at my destination when driving, especially when driving to work in the morning, since it was in the morning before work when my event occurred. So, each morning when I got to work, I'd call Carole. I also tried to keep her informed of anything going on with my body. It didn't help her if she thought I wasn't being candid. Then, she wouldn't trust me if I told her that nothing was wrong. What was interesting was that I found comforting her actually helped comfort me.

One thing that I unknowingly did that drove her crazy, though, was touching my chest. It was a reflex for me. Something I used to do even before my event. However, when Carole saw me do this, she immediately asked, "Is something wrong?" I understood her fear, so it didn't bother me, even though this happened quite often.

[*Side note: Looking back, I should have gone to see a doctor about my emotional health. Many in my support group did. I'm not sure why I didn't. It wasn't that I was averse to counseling or taking anti-anxiety medication (I had done that years ago for a totally separate issue). I think that, initially, it was because I had convinced myself that since I was going to die soon, my feelings were justified. So, instead of spending any effort on comforting myself, I concentrated on more important issues. Later, as the days and weeks passed, and the intensity of my anxiety began to diminish, I told myself that things might be getting better, so all I needed to do was wait a bit longer, that I would be okay if I gave it more time. So, for a while, I trudged through many days of doom and gloom, to the point where it had become a part of me. Eventually, when it appeared that my condition might be stabilizing, and with support from Carole, I allowed myself to think otherwise, that there may be hope. Not full-blown "All will be right" hope. More of "This doesn't have to be a death sentence" concession. I began to accept my condition, that it was something I could live with. And that lessened my fears. Another thing that helped me through my turmoil was going back to work. Besides being a great distraction, I felt my life returning to normal. Getting back to doing the things you enjoy and define you is a real boost. Don't get me wrong,*

I still had anxiety, but it was finally becoming manageable. However, as I know now, if I had sought help back when I needed it the most, I would have gotten to a better place sooner, and it would have saved me many restless nights.]

Doctor Visits

I was amazed at the number of doctor visits I had for one reason or another. Not everything was because of my dissection, though. Between my cardiologist, interventional cardiologist, cardiac surgeon, nephrologist, gastroenterologist, neurologist, neuro-ophthalmologist, ENT, and my GP doctor, my schedule was quite full. Plus, there were many tests and procedures – MRAs, stress tests, endoscopies, pulling my PEG tube out, eye exams, stent implant, and just plain old yearly exams. And finally, there were the extra hospital stays that I'll talk about later.

Several of these visits meant going back to Houston Methodist Hospital. I didn't mind going back to the hospital. Being there was actually kind of comforting, a sense of security. Carole, however, hated it, as I could imagine. To her, it was a reminder of some of the worse times in her life.

All of these doctor visits also meant using up all of my sick time at work. I hoped that I would not really get sick.

Aorta Dissection Support Group

Though Carole was and still is my greatest source of support, I needed more. Thankfully, I found some solace and hope in the *Aortic Dissection Support Group* on Facebook. In this group there are many survivors and loved ones of survivors. Some of these survivors have had several years since their dissection, some more than twenty years. And they were still going and still coping. This gave me renewed hope, hope that someday I would be just as much a warrior in this fight for survival as they are.

But besides the obvious support, one of the reasons that this group became so important to me was that it provided real accounts of survivor longevity, for many statistics on aorta dissection morbidity didn't take into account people's age, their health, their circumstances, and any new medical technology. Again, the Internet could be useful, but it could also be very misleading.

Plus, the support group provided me a sounding board for issues and questions that I might have. Finally, there was the comfort knowing that I was not alone in this struggle. I recommend support groups to anyone experiencing trauma in their life.

I would also like to mention another group called *Aortic Hope*. They spread awareness about aortic dissections as well as provide support to those in need.

John Ritter Foundation for Aortic Health

I would be remiss not to mention the John Ritter Foundation for Aortic Health. John Ritter was an actor, best known for his starring role in the 1970s' TV sitcom *Three's Company*, who died from an aortic dissection in 2003 at the age of fifty-four. He had gone to the hospital after experiencing chest pains. He was initially misdiagnosed as having a heart attack, which may have contributed to his death. Hours later, the correct diagnosis was made, but it was too late. Regardless, his death brought much-needed attention to this unheard-of disease, highlighting the need for awareness by the medical community.

As the foundation's statement explains, the organization is focused on "genetic research, widespread education, and radical advocacy" to alleviate "unnecessary suffering caused by the devastating lack of aortic awareness." The organization also came up with the "Ritter Rules" to help recognize an aortic dissection. They are a great resource for anyone wishing to learn more about aortic health.

Because of their genetic research initiative, I went to their Houston location for free genetic screening. This was to not only see if my dissection was caused by genetics, but also to alert my family members in case it was. The only problem with their screening is that they may or may not conduct research using your DNA. So, you would only hear back from them if they decided to use your DNA. I guess they did not use my DNA since I never heard back. I never did go and pay for getting the DNA test done myself, because after going over my screening questionnaire with them, it looked like I did not have any of the common indicators that my dissection was due to genetics (such as a family history of aortic disease; or connective tissue disorder symptoms like flexible joints, tendon/muscle rupture, long arms or legs, scoliosis, chest caves in or out, or easy bruising).

CHAPTER 13: One Year Out

It was now one full year after my event. August 2nd became my new birthday, my rebirth, so to speak. It was cause for celebration, time to take a moment and put things in perspective. I was still here, another year that I was lucky to have had. It was my Aortaversary, a new term I learned from my support group.

~~~~~~~~~~~~

To acknowledge those involved in saving my life, I created handwritten thank-you notes to St. John Hospital ER, Houston Methodist's Hospital CCU, Dr. Reardon, and Dr. Zoghbi. It was a small gesture, but I wanted them to know how appreciative I was for saving my life, giving me extra time in this world.

I also visited Methodist's CCU, at least from the outside. I tried to think back and imagine my time there, trying to remember what I saw, but those images were now vague. Considering the shape I was in and all the drugs, I wasn't sure what was real anyway. I wished I could have gone back inside, but it wasn't allowed.

In response to my thank-you note to St. John Hospital, someone from their Public Relations office called and asked me if I would be willing to be in an advertisement for St. John Hospital. I was, especially since I wished to promote knowledge about aortic dissections. I talked with one of their writers, and after getting Carole's and my picture taken in front of the hospital, I was
~~~~~~~~~~~~

pleasantly surprised to see my story in a few local publications. And it was also kind of nice when I got recognition from others who read the article.

~~~~~~~~~~~~

It was also time for my follow-up MRA. This is something that I would be doing yearly, to see if there were any changes, to see if another aneurysm was growing. I had tried to think positively about this, but considering there are no symptoms for an aneurysm, there was nothing to indicate one way or another how my health was really doing. Thankfully, my weird chest pains and discomforts had subsided somewhat, which lessened my worry, and I was getting used to certain pains that I now attributed to something other than my aorta. To me, it seemed that my dissection may have stabilized. But I knew that was just my blind optimism, as there was no way to really know without a medical scan if my dissection was okay or if it had worsened. Regardless, I clung to the hope that since my symptoms had waned, that I might have gotten better.

As the day approached to perform my MRA, I began to get nervous. Besides worrying about the test results, I was also starting to freak out about the actual procedure. My claustrophobia was getting the better of me, and I started imagining all sorts of possible weird things that might happen. One of the main fears was that the squeeze ball to signal the operators wouldn't work, and since I would be unable to get out of the machine on my own, I'd be trapped. Aaahhh! Stupid gerbils.

As luck would have it, just before my procedure, Hurricane Harvey hit the Houston area, causing havoc. Carole and I were lucky that we were not impacted by the storm. However, many in Houston were, and I was afraid that I would have to reschedule my MRA. I called Methodist Hospital and they said that they were still open. In fact, when Carole and I got to the hospital for my procedure, I was
~~~~~~~~~~~~

able to get my test done early as many others had canceled due to the hurricane.

This time, my MRA took two and a half hours. That was two and a half hours of being encased inside a very tight enclosure! Again, I am claustrophobic. So, being stuck in this MRA machine that long was a real challenge. In one of my earlier MRAs, the operators told me that putting a cloth over my eyes might help (a mind game where not actually seeing yourself inside makes it less real). To me it did help. So, just like the last time, I asked the operators to again cover my eyes with a cloth. However, this time, because of the extended duration, I had to really work on keeping myself from getting panicky.

The test went well. But apparently there was some confusion about whether the test was complete enough. The test orders only requested a Thoracic Aorta MRA. I knew that I also needed my Abdominal Aorta examined. (Another example of always looking out for yourself.) So, the operators agreed with me, and they said that they would work it out with Dr. Reardon. They were not concerned, because as they told me, certain doctors had *privileges*. It was good to have such a respected doctor on your team.

Later that same day, I met with Dr. Reardon to go over my MRA results. My nerves were on edge again. I eagerly awaited to hear the results, but at the same time I dreaded them as well. Well, things turned out good. Dr. Reardon told me that there were no changes to my aorta over the last year, which meant there were no new aneurysms. Dr. Reardon seemed pleased, which made me feel good. He also told me that if my aorta remained stable, that maybe in a year or two I could extend my examinations to every two or even three years. That gave me a lot of hope.

~~~~~~~~~~~~~
~~~~~~~~~~~~~

So, looking back over the past year was a little surreal for me. I still found it hard to believe that what I went through was real. In fact, a part of me still wanted to believe that it didn't happen.

Regardless, I was greatly relieved that I was stable, and that gave me more confidence in that I wouldn't die in the very near future. But I still cringed whenever I felt something odd in my chest. My goal now was to try to quickly quiet those gerbils from letting my imagination run wild. If I could do that, then maybe I could return to a more normal.

CHAPTER 14: Second Year

Fainting Spells

Nearly a year from my event, I began to experience these near-fainting spells; at least that was what they most felt like. This would happen several times, every now and then. Plus, they would come on randomly.

The first time one of these spells occurred was after eating lunch at a Chinese restaurant. I was on my way back to work, driving my car and listening to music. When I turned a corner, I instantly got severely light-headed. I thought I was going to pass out, so I slowed down and frantically looked for a safe place to pull over. Before I could reach a turn-off from the road, the feeling dissipated. It lasted only a couple of seconds, but it felt much longer. It scared the hell out of me. I didn't think too much of it, other than being thankful that I didn't actually pass out. I wondered why this just happened. I could only think that maybe it was my inner ear being affected by sinus pressure, because I had been having sinus issues for a while. So, I attributed it to that.

It would be weeks later before I experienced my second episode, and over the next three years I would randomly have more spells. All came on instantly, all lasted only a couple seconds or so, and all felt like I would pass out. Luckily, I never did.

Worried, I tried to examine what might have been connected to these episodes. From what I remembered, each time, I had sinus issues and was listening to music. In fact, part of me started thinking that maybe the music was triggering these episodes. That was because as I started to become faint, the music seemed to become very prominent in my head. My reasoning was that the music was affecting my inner ear, which was affected by sinus pressure. Oh, there was one more coincidence. For all but one episode, I had just been eating a meal.

Besides my first episode, there was only one more episode while driving, and like the first time, it only lasted for a couple of seconds. These episodes were scary enough on their own, but what really concerned me was driving. So far, I hadn't passed out, but maybe that was because I had just been extremely lucky. However, the thought of giving up driving was equally as scary.

Plus, now that I was paranoid about it, any feeling I got in my head made me panicky and I started feeling dizzy. It became so that I didn't know any more whether what I was experiencing was real or self-induced. Either way, I became very conscious of myself and where I was driving. I kept a constant vigil of where I could pull off the road, just in case. I dreaded driving on the highway or anywhere that was far away.

Other episodes included a visit to the dentist's office, and a couple of times at a restaurant. At the dentist's office, I was sitting waiting for my appointment. When I went to get up, the spell came on. Again, there was music playing in the waiting room, and it was not too long after having eaten breakfast. This time, I began wondering if this was due to a change in position. Maybe something to do with my BP medications?

At the restaurants, I was out with Carole, her brother, and his fiancée. Both incidents occurred during the same weekend, and I had just caught a head cold. At the first restaurant, the episode occurred after just having sat down for dinner. There was music playing in the background, and all of a sudden, I got that light-headed feeling. I sat there trying my best to stay focused and not pass out. Carole and the others, however, looked at me and thought I was having a stroke. They became extremely scared for me. I told them what happened, but Carole still requested that I go through some of the standard exercises to check for a stroke. Thankfully, I did not exhibit any of the signs.

The next day, at the second restaurant, we had just finished lunch, and we were standing around inside the restaurant talking. When a new song began to play in the background (I was almost positive it was the same song that I heard the night before when I experienced my earlier spell), I again felt like I might pass out, but this time it was not as extreme. I didn't feel like it was imminent that I might pass out. I told Carole that I needed to leave – NOW! I told her that the music was bothering me. And, as soon as I stepped out of the restaurant and away from the music, I at once felt normal. It may just have been a coincidence, but this convinced me that the music was at least part of what was triggering my spells. Little did I know.

Here's where I caution others not to do as I did. I was initially hesitant going to the doctor for fear that they would tell me not to drive. However, after several episodes, I conceded that I needed to do something. So, I started with my GP doctor, Dr. Janoe. I asked him if my sinuses could cause me to become dizzy. I also told him that I had been having a lot of sinus pressure. He said it could be possible, so he sent me for a head MRI. The MRI results came back normal – thank God. He then had me follow up with an ENT – Dr. Yoon. I asked Dr. Yoon if my sinuses or inner ear could be causing me to become light-headed. She didn't think so. She said that what I was describing was usually a cardiac issue. But she did notice that I had an inner ear infection. So, she prescribed me an antibiotic, a fluoroquinolone, the same type of drug that might have caused my dissection. At first, I refused it, fearing that I could cause further damage to my aorta. (I would continue to refuse taking any fluoroquinolone in the future.) But Dr. Yoon said that since I would be using such a small topical dose, it wouldn't be a concern. So, for this particular treatment, I relented in using it. In response, my inner ear infection cleared up, and even though Dr. Yoon did not hold the same opinion, I was hopeful that this might resolve my near-fainting spells. Again, little did I know.

Indigestion?

Also around the start of my second year, I began to experience indigestion when I walked. At least I attributed my symptoms to indigestion since the discomfort in my chest felt like a large gas bubble. The pain wasn't severe, but it was worrisome. I also noticed that I only got the pain from walking, never from upper body exercise or any other physical exertion. Plus, the pain seemed to coincide after having had a large or *bad* meal. But the final thought in my reasoning was that the pain started about five minutes into my walking and then stopped after about twenty minutes of continuous walking. If this was cardiac, wouldn't the pain continue? This rationalization would prevent me from seeking medical evaluation. For the time being.

Ischemia

Well, it would turn out that I was wrong about my indigestion. After several weeks of experiencing indigestion, I eventually mentioned to my cardiologist, Dr. Zoghbi, that I wished to try to reduce my Metoprolol from 200 mg a day. As I mentioned before, I had read online that Metoprolol could worsen digestive issues, and I was hoping that by reducing the Metoprolol, my indigestion issues would likewise be reduced. Seemed logical to me.

However, Dr. Zoghbi wasn't so sure. Being cautious, he first ordered me a stress test, another nuclear stress test using Regadenoson to artificially race my heart. It was the same type of test I had done previously in the hospital. And I hated this test as much as before, that feeling like your heart is racing uncontrollably.

Regardless, the test did not show anything abnormal, as I had expected.

What I didn't know at the time, though, was that Dr. Zoghbi was concerned with something called ST segments on my EKGs. These ST segments had him convinced that all was not well, so he ordered me a different type of stress test. This stress test would require more exertion.

It was now April of 2018, well into the second year of my event, when I had this new stress test. While lying on my back, I pedaled a bicycle-type device that got harder to pedal as time went on. Unfortunately (or fortunately, since I needed to find out what was really going on), this test came back abnormal. It showed that my heart was not getting enough oxygen to handle the physical demand. Apparently, this suggested that I had some type of ischemia. And, from my EKG, this ischemia appeared to be caused by my Left Main Artery. Crap!

Knowing that my Left Main Artery had been compromised from my surgery (fifty percent stenosis), Dr. Zoghbi brought in an interventional cardiologist – Dr. Colin Barker. Dr. Barker informed me that he suspected that my Left Main Artery got "kinked" when reattached onto my aorta and scar tissue had most likely built up. He said that he had seen this before. The next step would be to have an angiogram done to see the extent of my blockage and get a better view of where the blockage lay. To do so, Dr. Barker needed to perform a heart catheterization. But, because I had chronic kidney disease, he would need to use much less contrast than normal because the contrast could damage my kidneys further.

Dr. Barker told me that most likely I would need to have a stent put in place to straighten out my artery, and, if need be, that he'd do it when he performed the catheterization. The stent would be a drug-eluting stent, meaning that it was coated with medication to reduce the chance of clotting around the stent. The bad news with having this type of stent was that I would need to be put on a blood thinner for a year instead of six months.

A final piece of information – Dr. Barker informed me that because of my dissected and weakened aorta, it was risky to perform the catheterization via the artery through my leg (which currently was the most common place to insert a catheterization line). Instead, he would use the artery in my arm, which would then bypass my aorta. This was a newer method that Dr. Barker was skilled in. Again, I felt very lucky to have such great physicians available to me.

Needless to say, both Carole and I were stunned and worried. I truthfully did not think that I had any severe issue since I was not experiencing any other symptoms – like shortness of breath and fatigue. But Dr. Barker talked like this would be a straightforward procedure. He had the same confidence that Dr. Reardon gave Carole, which went a long way in soothing our anxiety.

But we still had a few questions. We were told that the procedure would not take long, maybe an hour or two. And, normally, this would be done as an outpatient procedure. But, because of my kidneys, Dr. Barker wanted me to stay overnight in the hospital for observation. Plus, to help my kidneys, he would have my kidneys flushed afterwards. This was supposed to reduce any potential damage that may result from the contrast used. After the procedure, Dr. Barker said that I should be able to resume normal activities in a few days. But until then, I would need to take it easy. Well, it didn't sound too bad, but anytime someone starts poking around inside your arteries, you tend to get scared. After all, one scrape or poke too hard and you could have a serious problem.

Once Dr. Barker finished talking with us, Dr. Zoghbi returned. He warned me that I was to absolutely forgo any more physical exertion until I got my artery fixed. Considering how long I had been exercising with this condition, I couldn't believe how lucky I had been. Every time I thought about it, I cringed. God certainly had watched over me. Oh, and one more thing, Dr. Zoghbi told me that I needed to schedule my procedure as soon as possible. That solidified how critical things were. So, before leaving, I scheduled my procedure for the very next Friday.

Well, as Carole and I headed home, we were now in a state of fear. My dissection nightmare just kept going.

Stent

During the next few days before my procedure, Carole and I got even more anxious. Not just from why I needed the procedure, but also from having the procedure. Besides the risks the procedure involved, we still didn't know for sure the extent of my condition. The only good thing was that we looked forward to putting this next obstacle behind us.

Since I would be spending the night, I didn't want Carole making that horrendous drive back and forth to the hospital again by herself. So, I convinced her to spend the night in the Marriott hotel that was across the street from the hospital. In fact, there was a sky bridge that connected the hotel with the hospital. I could see the relief on her face.

It was finally Friday, April 27th, 2018. On the morning of my procedure, Carole and I went to the hospital early. I registered and began my pre-op. Prior to coming to the hospital, I had blood work drawn as part of my pre-op. I was told that my potassium level was high (5.9, normal is below 5.2). Dr. Barker wanted to do another test to recheck my potassium. While waiting for the new test results, they got me prepped. An IV was started (after several attempts at finding my vein, including digging around with the needle – Ughh!), and they shaved my right arm where Dr. Barker would insert the catheter.

After a while, Dr. Barker came by. He said that my potassium level was still too high (now at 6.3), and he thought it was too risky to perform the catheterization today. So, unfortunately, he told me that I needed to reschedule. Next time, though, he wanted me to spend the night before in the hospital so that they could flush my kidneys with fluids to bring my potassium down. So, without any recourse, I thanked Dr. Barker for his cautiousness, and I rescheduled my procedure for the following Friday. After getting all psyched up, both Carole and I felt disappointed and even more anxious. We both had hoped to have gotten this over with. But instead, we would have to wait another week.

One highlight of the cancellation was that Carole's hotel room was already booked and could not be canceled. So, we decided to make the best out of a bad situation and stay at the hotel anyway. But first, dinner out at a nice Italian restaurant called Prego, and then a wonderful breakfast at the hotel. Sort of a mini getaway. A fun venture except for the pressing thought of my pending stent and the worry that something very bad could happen while waiting. The only other drawback was that we would be booking the hotel yet again for the next week.

Well, the next Thursday came, the day before my procedure. (Luckily, without exercising, I had not experienced any more "indigestion" feelings.) When I got to the hospital this time, I needed to register as in-patient to the hospital. I thought it would be relatively quick, but it took a few hours for them to find me a bed (even for such a huge hospital as Methodist, they could be quite busy). Luckily, Carole and I were already used to waiting in the hospital. Though, we both started getting a little impatient for the delay.

I finally got to my room, and they eventually got me hooked up to an IV to start my fluids. Part of being back in a hospital room felt eerily familiar, but part of this stay was different. Maybe because of the difference in criticality. Or maybe it was because I was not on any strong pain medications. My only major concern was trying to take my normal daily medications – at my normal daily time. Apparently, hospitals did not accommodate patients' personal medication schedules. So, I hoped that I could take all my medications within limits.

Carole stayed with me for most of the day, but she soon tired. With the hotel nearby, she headed back to her room, only a short walk away. Even with her gone, I felt better knowing she was close by.

The night went as expected. Not much sleep and waking up early to be poked for more blood work. Carole came in with coffee and a muffin in hand. It's nice having a Starbucks in the hospital lobby.

Soon, I was carted back off to the cardiology procedure room. And, as the previous week, I got prepped all over again. This time, I was told that my potassium level was within range (4.5). So, my procedure was a go!

Dr. Barker arrived and informed me that he would be performing my procedure using robotics. Neat! He asked me if I would be willing for the hospital to tape my procedure so it could be used for training and such. I told him that was fine with me. So, someone from the hospital came to have me sign authorization papers. I found it all interesting.

It wasn't long before they wheeled me away to the procedure room. I said goodbye to Carole. Both she and I were nervous.

In the procedure room, one of the technicians asked what kind of music I would like to hear. I answered AC/DC. In a few minutes, I was hearing AC/DC playing away. Cool!

As I was lying there waiting, I was surprised to find myself feeling semi-relaxed. I didn't understand why, considering the previous anxiety. I was eventually told that I would be given a couple of medications to put me in a semi-conscious state. Semi-conscious? Wow! That surprised me and caused me a bit of concern. However, once they started the medications, I remembered nothing.

Next thing I knew, I awoke in the recovery room. Carole was there and I felt fine. I was told the procedure went well. I was also told that the blockage in my Left Main Artery was over ninety percent. Both Carole and I were flabbergasted. That was extremely dangerous.

When I looked at my arm where the catheter was inserted, I saw that it was bruised and quite swollen. A compression bandage was currently wrapped around it, not only to keep the swelling down, but to also help stop the bleeding from the catheterization insertion hole. This was needed because I had been started on Brilinta, a strong blood thinner.

Later, the nurse took the compression bandage off. There was no bleeding, but my arm was still very swollen. They said that it was most likely due to the Brilinta. The nurse spent a lot of time massaging my arm, trying to push the swollen blood away. A few hours later, I headed back to my room. Not unexpectedly, Dr. Barker wanted me to spend another night in the hospital for observation. It also meant another night for Carole in the hotel.

The only issue that arose during the night was that I began to experience a fast heart rate. An EKG was ordered, but nothing critical was seen. I thought that I was merely having a panic attack.

The next morning came, and after a few more tests, including another EKG, I was sent home. I was told to be careful over the next couple of days. I wasn't sure if I was relieved or not. I tried not to think about what I had just gone through. Again, I just wanted all of this to be over.

TIA

For the first few days after my stent procedure, I felt fine. To take it easy, I took a few days off work. Then, on the fifth day since my surgery, a Wednesday, Carole left home to go to a luncheon with her friends. I felt fine and didn't think much about it.

So, I was at my desk playing a video game, and I started feeling light-headed. And like before, the music in the game became intense. I quickly got up and headed to the bedroom. That was the last thing I remember.

Later, Carole returned home from her lunch. I heard her frantically calling for me, asking me what happened. I had just awakened in the bedroom. I was lying on the bed. I got up and headed towards her. She asked me again what happened, and I looked at her blankly. I saw that she was scared, but I couldn't comprehend why. She then asked me about the blood. Blood? What blood? She pointed to my arms. I looked down and saw that my arms were cut and bloody, the blood having already dried. Gently, she told me to sit. She then told me that she thought that I may have had a stroke. I was still not comprehending, but I sensed her fear. She asked me to look at her, but when I did, I apparently did not look directly at her even though I thought I was. Really concerned now, she had me do all the checks for stroke, like smile, raise my arms, and speak. I could do those things, but I was still trying to clear my head and understand what happened. For some reason, I couldn't think clearly.

Becoming even more scared, Carole called our friend Allyson, the one who worked in the ER. Allyson told Carole that I most likely had a TIA, and I would most likely be okay. She also told Carole that she and her husband, Jerry, would be right over to take us to the hospital.

As we waited for our friends to drive over, Carole showed me what she first saw when she came home. In our foyer, there was broken glass and blood all over. When Carole first saw the mess, she thought maybe our cat, Pippin, had jumped onto our cabinet and knocked off some vases and figurines. Instead, as we would deduce later, I must have fallen into the cabinet and then against the wall. Because, besides the blood on the wall, one of the nearby walls was banged up. Dumbfounded, I told her that I had no memory of it. She then had me get ready to head to the hospital. I headed into our bathroom and looked in the mirror. I couldn't believe what I saw. It looked like I had been in a fierce fight. What the hell happened to me? I was very confused. What was also odd is that I didn't feel any pain.

Later, Carole would also find blood on our bed, on the bathroom sink, and on the medicine cabinet. There was also a bottle of saline nasal spray with blood on it. Just what I was trying to do will forever remain a mystery. To this day, I have no recollection of the event.

Allyson and Jerry soon arrived, and they drove us to St. John Hospital in Nassau Bay. Allyson gave Carole a lot of hope that everything would be okay. By this time, I was finally beginning to have clearer thoughts. Or at least I thought I was.

When we got to the hospital, Carole explained to the doctor what had happened. The hospital immediately responded in case I had a stroke. Many tests were run including a head MRI. I remember being asked what year it was. I could not answer the question and I began to cry. The mounting frustration began to take its toll.

Well, the doctor didn't think I had a stroke either, but I would need to stay in the hospital for observation. As it would turn out, they would keep me for two nights, much to the dislike of both Carole and me. Many more tests were run, including something called a bubble test (tiny bubbles were injected into my vein to check if there were any tiny holes between my heart chambers).

To give full disclosure, I told the doctor about my past episodes where I had gotten light-headed to the point that I thought I might faint. I explained that each episode had been after hearing music and that I was having sinus/ear congestion. A neurologist was called in who wondered if I might have a form of epilepsy, and that my episodes may have been seizures. A new test was run where I had some type of head gear strapped on. The head gear looked very sci-fi-ish. It had electrodes all over it to monitor my brain activity. They then had me listen to music to see if anything triggered a response.

No response. Either my episodes were completely random, or I just didn't have the right trigger, or maybe it was just not neurological.

After the second night and more tests ordered, Carole and I began to wonder if the hospital was just keeping me there to run unneeded tests, especially since I had good insurance and my deductible was already met. It got to the point that I told the charge nurse that I would be leaving with or without their permission. I was finally allowed to leave.

When I got home, I surveyed the foyer again to try to regain some sort of memory of what happened. But it was useless. Either those memory cells are gone, or I was never really conscious to begin with. Carole told me she spent a lot of time cleaning up the place, especially trying to get the blood off our bed's comforter. The only marks left were a chipped crystal bowl and a gouge in the wall. Of course, there were a couple of items now missing off the cabinet.

The whole experience put me and Carole on edge. Again, another life-threatening event, out of the blue with no warning. Just when I was beginning to feel more confident about my health and my future, this event now made Carole and me fearful about being left alone. (And I don't dare play video games alone in the house even to this day.) I also wondered if it would ever be safe enough for me to drive. I shuddered at the thought of if my TIA had happened while driving. When would this nightmare end?

Nosebleeds

Well, things settled down for the next couple of months. Just in time for my next adventure. Woo-hoo!

Ever since I went on Brilinta, I found out three things – I bruised easily, I bled easily, and I got chronic nosebleeds – a trifecta! The nosebleeds were not that terrible, but they did take much longer to stop than before I was on Brilinta. In fact, it got to the point that I contemplated going to my ENT to see about getting the veins in my nose cauterized. Little did I know that that decision would be made for me.

At the end of July 2018, on a Friday, I woke up, showered, and got dressed as normal. Then, as was common for me, I blew my nose due to congestion built up during the night. This caused my left nasal passage to start bleeding. Again, nothing too bad. Just a constant small bleed. Thinking that it would eventually stop, I went about my business.

Well, after several hours of trying various methods to stop the bleeding, Carole and I decided that maybe it was best to go get my nose cauterized. It was too late to get in to see my ENT, so I first tried one of those urgent care places. Well, apparently, they don't cauterize nosebleeds. They said I needed to go to the ER. So, assuming that this would be something simple, I decided to go to a new local hospital, University of Texas Medical Branch (UTMB), which was close to my house.

I saw one of UTMB's ER doctors and explained my medical history leading me to my current situation. Before resorting to cauterization, the ER doctor wanted to first spray a nasal decongestant in my nose. This was supposed to narrow the blood vessels in my nose in an attempt to help stop the bleeding. Normally, I wouldn't use a nasal decongestant since it could raise my blood pressure. However, this was for medical necessity, and the ER doctor didn't expect that it would have much effect on my BP anyway. Well, the nose spray didn't work. Next, the ER doctor wanted me to squeeze my nose for at least fifteen minutes to see if that helped. That didn't work either. So, the ER doctor finally decided to cauterize my nose using silver nitrate.

It had been a long time since I had my nose cauterized. The last time being about fifty years ago as a kid. I forgot just how much that stuff burned. Nothing excruciating, but definitely a discomfort. Especially since this doctor apparently wasn't adept in using silver nitrate and just slathered it on way up into my nasal passage – multiple times! The first attempt of silver nitrate did nothing. Neither did the second. Or the third. Or the fourth. Finally, on the fifth attempt and after a large amount of silver nitrate, my nose stopped bleeding. The ER doctor said that if the bleeding returned, the next option would be to pack my nose until I could get in to see my ENT.

Carole and I headed home, hoping that the bleeding had stopped for good. At home, I went to take a look in the mirror. Carole had told me that my nose looked bad, but it wasn't until I saw my nose that I understood just how bad. All around the tip and the inside of my nose was black from the silver nitrate. My nose looked like it was charred in a fire. Well, at least there was no blood.

Things remained stable, so Carole and I eventually headed to bed. As chance would have it, Carole's daughter, Jennifer, along with Jennifer's new boyfriend, Stitz, came in to visit for the same weekend, and they arrived a little before midnight on Friday. Carole and I got up from out of bed to greet them. Apparently, the act of getting up and moving around agitated the pressure on my nose and the bleeding restarted. However, this time, the bleeding was more profuse. Scared, I knew I had to return to the ER.

Besides having her daughter at home, Carole was extremely tired from all of the earlier stress. She asked if it was okay if she stayed home. She already knew what the ER was going to do next – pack my nose. So, I told her to get some rest, that I could handle it alone. My only problem was, what could I use to stuff my nose to stop the bleeding so I could drive? After having seen this done in a movie, Carole suggested a tampon. After a few jokes and a few laughs, I soon relented, thinking "What the hell?" I was thinking that this might be a little embarrassing going to the ER with a tampon sticking out my nose, but what turned out to be even more humorous was that Carole needed to get the tampon from our guest bathroom, which was currently occupied. Carole hoped that it was Jennifer in the bathroom. It wasn't. It was Jennifer's new boyfriend, who we just met for the first time. So, Carole waited for Stitz to leave before going in. She didn't tell him then that she needed to get a tampon (for me!), but she did relate the story the next day. If that wasn't embarrassing, I don't know what is. So, after stuffing this tampon as best I could up my small nostril, I headed back to the ER. By this time, it was around 1 a.m.

So, on my second visit to the UTMB Hospital ER, I again had to relate my story of what led me here. The new ER doctor agreed that packing my nose was best. Now, I had been thinking that this packing would be some type of gauze-like material that they would merely shove up my nose, something similar to the tampon I currently had in, but something designed for the nose. What I didn't realize was this packing, or "tampon," as it was actually called, was an inflatable device. Plus, the doctor first had to shove the packing way up into my sinus, not just into my nostril, much further than what I would have thought possible. And the pain? Well, when they told me to take a deep breath and try to relax, I should had known that this would be painful. On a scale of one to ten, I'd say this was a good seven. But this wasn't the end of it. Then, the doctor proceeded to inflate the packing. Another round of pain. And, to top things off, a tube hangs off the end of the packing and out my nose, which would be used later to remove it. The doctor taped the end of the tube on my face to keep it in place and out of the way. I couldn't wait to see myself in the mirror with a tampon string hanging out my nose. I'd laugh at it all except that having this packing jammed way up into my sinus was more than a constant major discomfort. It was downright painful. The doctor prescribed me some minor painkillers and told me where there was a twenty-four-hour pharmacy open. So, I headed to the pharmacy at about 3:00 a.m.

I got home and showed off my new face to Carole. That brought more joking about having a tampon string hanging out of my blackened nose. I'm glad now that no one thought about taking a picture. But this did cause both of us to worry a little about how I would look when we went out in public. Maybe some makeup? Maybe a lot of makeup. Anyway, that issue would have to wait until tomorrow. At the moment, I was too exhausted and in too much pain. All I wished to do now was go to bed.

The next day, Saturday, started off with my nose still hurting from the packing. The constant pressure and pain built up over time. The painkillers that the ER doctor prescribed me weren't helping. So, I ended up sitting in a chair, not feeling very sociable with our guests. After a while, the pain became unbearable. It wasn't that the pain was so intense, but after hours of it, my pain threshold seemed to weaken. I told Carole that I needed to go back to the ER and see if they could give me something stronger for the pain.

Again, with Carole's daughter in town, she asked if I needed her to go with me. I said no. So, back to the UTMB Hospital ER for the third time in less than twenty-four hours. Once again, I told my entire story, and explained that the pain was too much for the minor pain medicine given me. The ER doctor definitely understood how nasal packing could be unbearable. So, she first asked if I could have someone drive me home. I replied yes, that I could call my wife. So, to mitigate the pain, she gave me morphine. To my surprise, the morphine didn't touch the pain. Fearful that I would just have to stay in pain, the ER doctor told me not to worry, that she would try fentanyl next. Luckily, the fentanyl dimmed the pain to a tolerable level. The ER doctor then prescribed me a more potent pain medication for home. By this time, Carole arrived to drive me home. Both of us were glad that I was finally starting to feel better. I couldn't believe the trauma I had been through all due to a stupid nosebleed. Unfortunately, my trauma was not at an end.

~~~~~~~~~~~~~
~~~~~~~~~~~~~

The earliest that I could make an appointment with my ENT, Dr. Yoon, was for Tuesday. By the time I saw her, it had been three days since my nose was packed. I was thinking that surely the bleeding had stopped by now. I mean, I hadn't noticed any bleeding, either from my nose or in the back of my mouth. So, when Dr. Yoon carefully removed the packing, to my surprise, my nose was still bleeding.

Dr. Yoon examined my nose but could not find the source of my bleeding. She then attempted to perform more cauterization with silver nitrate. Being more skilled at this than the ER doctor, she didn't just slather it on. However, the silver nitrate wasn't working for her either.

Dr. Yoon informed me that there were two options left – one, she could electro-cauterize my nose by performing nasal surgery, or two, she could refer me to a specialist who could insert a stent-like device into the end of the sphenopalatine artery of my nose, acting like a plug. Option two was much riskier, because they would have had to perform a catheterization through one of my main arteries, more than likely having to go into my femoral artery and up through my aorta. Considering the weakened state of my aorta due to my dissection, I went with option one. Dr. Yoon scheduled my surgery for later that day at Clear Lake Regional Hospital. This would be my fourth hospital in a span of about three months. Not the kind of achievement that I was shooting for.

To get me in for surgery today, Dr. Yoon had me go to the ER immediately after my visit with her. At first, I felt a little embarrassed having to get "emergency" surgery for a nosebleed, but there wasn't a good alternative. So, after some blood work and a couple of hours wait, I was finally prepped for surgery. Once Dr. Yoon came into the ER, I was given a sedative.

The next thing I knew was that I was in recovery gagging on something in my throat. Carole was there with Dr. Yoon as she explained that she could never pinpoint exactly where my nosebleed stemmed from, other than she saw blood seeping from somewhere in my sphenopalatine artery. The problem, though, was that I was still bleeding, and this time, the bleeding was even heavier. With the amount of blood flowing down my throat, I was really scared. Why wasn't this stopping? What else could they do? To keep me from swallowing too much blood, they used a suction hose down my throat. Carole told me that she was scared to see so much blood being siphoned off. There was a storage container behind me that Carole said was filling quickly. Dr. Yoon said that the blood was really a mixture of mucous and blood, so that the volume wasn't as bad as it looked. Well, that was easy for her to say, not being her blood gushing down the back of her throat. However, I wasn't too happy. Neither was Carole. Things were actually better before my surgery. Why was everything the doctors doing making things worse? Unfortunately, Dr. Yoon knew she had to put me back under for a second surgery and try to cauterize even more of my sinus.

Before leaving for surgery again, Carole noticed that my blood pressure was dangerously high; my systolic was near 180. That was too high for someone even without a dissection, but for me it could be devastating. Because I did not have a chance to go home today, I was unable to take my evening medications. I was too out of it from the anesthesia to really think about it, but Carole was there, yet again, to look out for me. She told Dr. Yoon that my blood pressure was dangerously too high. Dr. Yoon agreed and ordered me something to bring my blood pressure down. After I received some blood pressure medication, I was hauled off back to surgery.

Well, in this case, the second time was a charm. Dr. Yoon was able to stop the bleeding. However, I would have to spend the night in the hospital for observation.

~~~~~~~~~~~~~
~~~~~~~~~~~~~

Since my nosebleeds were attributed to being on Brilinta, Dr. Yoon communicated with my cardiologist, Dr. Zoghbi, about switching me to Plavix instead. Plavix still had an increased risk of nosebleeds, but not as bad. As I told Dr. Zoghbi later, Brilinta was very good about keeping my blood from clotting, probably too good.

So, whether it was due to the cauterization or the switch to Plavix, my nosebleed problems dwindled. I would still get minor bleeding, but nothing like what necessitated surgery. I couldn't wait until I could get off of these anti-clotting agents.

In the meantime, all I could do was use saline washes and rinses to soothe my nose and sinuses. I also stopped all antihistamines as well as nasal steroid sprays that I had been using for allergies. After a while, I discovered that the saline rinses did as good a job in the long run.

Now, as with my dissected aorta, risk of ischemia, and risk of TIAs, I had also become ultra-paranoid about nosebleeds. This new normal sucked.

No More Fainting

After a while, I noticed that I hadn't had any near-fainting spells for a while. Unfortunately, as I began thinking why, Dr. Yoon may have been right – my near-fainting spells were most likely not due to an inner ear problem or my sinuses.

As I previously mentioned, I saw my cardiologist, Dr. Zoghbi, concerning my indigestion, which ultimately led to the discovery of my Left Main Artery blockage and stent. Well, ever since I had my stent implanted, I hadn't had a near-fainting spell. I've had some dizziness, but nothing to the point where I thought I may pass out. I was thinking that my recent dizziness was self-induced from my paranoia (usually when I was driving, listening to certain music, and feeling my sinus pressure change). Anyway, over the next few months, even this dizziness faded away.

So, I was guessing now that I had been very, very, VERY lucky in not passing out or even dying, because these spells may have been due to my Left Main Artery blockage. Looking back, it scared me to think that my blood flow had been so critical. I could have died any one of those times when I was about to pass out, or any of those times when I felt that indigestion feeling. I tried not to think about it, but then I told myself that God must have been there for me.

Oh, and one more thing that scared me about my ischemia. For our anniversary (which was only a couple of weeks before we found out about my ischemia), Carole and I went on a vacation to California. We spent a few days there in the wine country. To think that I was walking around all that time with such a life-threatening issue. I guess what they say is true – ignorance is bliss!

CHAPTER 15: Third Year

Two years went by, and I again celebrated my new birthday. The last time I celebrated I thought I could put the bad times behind me and move on with my life. Well, things didn't go as smoothly as I had hoped during the past year. Regardless, I was hoping that the next year would be better.

And…it was.

Things finally went smoothly, at least smoothly in that I didn't almost die, or have more surgeries, or more hospital stays, or more critical issues. It's all in one's perspective. Plus, my body continued to strengthen, which meant more stamina. I also experienced less pain, less discomfort. Though, that wasn't to say that I was never without some type of chest discomfort or weird feeling. I think I will have those feelings the rest of my life, whether they are real or figments of my paranoia. But, overall, I was feeling better, which reduced my anxiety and brought me hope.

Then, there was my yearly MRA. I still had claustrophobia (didn't matter how many times I had done this before, I still had to force myself not to freak out). I still worried about the results. But, afterwards, when I talked with my cardiac surgeon, Dr. Reardon...everything was still stable! Yay! First, I thanked God, and then I started thinking that maybe (fingers crossed), I might actually get to live to a reasonable old age. At least Dr. Reardon thought so.

He told me that he expected to keep seeing me for many years ahead (at least until he retired).

~~~~~~~~~~~~~

After hearing the good news of my MRA, I felt brave enough to finally venture on a trip overseas to France, much to the delight of Carole. I was still scared about being that far away, especially in a foreign country, but I was able to convince myself that, if I had survived for this long, I should be okay enough for a week away (even with the long flights where I'd be stuck for hours, over the ocean, with literally no way to quickly get to a hospital). I kept telling myself that I *probably* wouldn't have a crisis in that length of time. Of course, I still worried about where I'd be and if there was a major hospital nearby. But I was trying not to be overly paranoid. I wanted desperately to start having a more normal life. So, I tried my best to push aside my fears and just do it. Baby steps.

However, I did have one real concern – nosebleeds. I would still be on Plavix during the trip, and I was afraid of two things. First, would the pressurized, dry air of the plane trigger a nosebleed? And second, how would I handle a flourishing nosebleed in public? That would be embarrassing, to say the least, having people on the plane or on one of our tours eye me as I try not to bleed all over the place.

So, Carole and I bought these nosebleed pads online (again, they were really just nose tampons), and I asked my ENT doctor what else could I do. Dr. Yoon said that if I would get a nosebleed, I should soak a cotton ball in nasal decongestant spray and stuff it up my nose to narrow the artery and help restrict the blood flow. That and pinch my nose for twenty minutes. Similar to what the ER doctor had me do. Boy, did I hope nothing bad happened when around other people.

And, as it turned out...my trip was great! No nosebleeds. No medical issues. Nothing notable (from a health point of view). Plus, a trip to France held so many distractions that I didn't dwell (*much*) on my
~~~~~~~~~~~~~

condition. Not only did I enjoy this trip, it also made me more positive about doing future trips. Not that wherever I would go wouldn't need to be someplace that had immediate and good medical care. I wasn't that brave.

~~~~~~~~~~~~~

Soon after my trip to France, it was time for my semi-annual appointment with my cardiologist. It had also been one year now since my stent surgery, and I was eager to get off of Plavix. But Dr. Zoghbi was a bit conservative, and since I was currently not having any critical issues with my blood thinner, he thought it was safer for me to stay on Plavix for another year. I was a bit disappointed, but he was the expert, so I stayed on Plavix and hoped my nose would behave. As it turned out, this would be a good thing later.

Hearing Music

But, even with things getting better, weird things still happened.

The first weird issue was when I got a cold. Usually, when I got a head cold, my sinuses drained, causing all sorts of mucus buildup. And, with my throat muscle problems from my stroke, gagging and coughing and snoring became a problem, especially for Carole, who was trying to sleep next to me with all of this noise. So, when I had a bad night, I headed to the living room to sleep in my recliner chair.

What happened next was totally unexpected. It was summertime, and our air conditioner unit was running outside. As I lay there, trying to fall asleep, I could hear the hum of the AC unit. Then, I began to hear music. Now, when I say "hear" music, I mean real music, as if the radio was playing. At first, I was scared, thinking that I was becoming delirious again. But I soon noticed that the music was tuned to the humming of the AC unit. I looked up on the Internet and found articles stating that this was not that abnormal, just a way of someone's mind trying to make sense of background noise. I also thought that the severe sinus pressure I currently had
~~~~~~~~~~~~~

played into this. So, after calming myself down, I instead tried to enjoy the music. Eventually, I fell asleep.

Testosterone Replacement Therapy

The second weird issue was when I started having heart palpitations again. Out of the blue, I started experiencing random bouts of heart fluttering and pounding heartbeats. Nothing serious enough to go to the doctor, but enough to make me concerned. So, I started looking for anything that had recently happened or changed in my life. That was when I correlated my palpitations with my recent testosterone replacement therapy pellets, or really, my change in testosterone level. (As with a lot of men, getting older resulted in low testosterone for me. For more than a year prior to my event, the replacement therapy I had been using to boost my testosterone level was to have five to six small testosterone pellets about the size of a large grain of rice injected into the fat of one of my buttocks. These pellets would last about six months before dissolving. However, as commonly happens with hormone replacement therapy, my testosterone levels were on a roller-coaster ride, surging and ebbing with the rise and fall of the pellets' strength.) Again, researching this on the Internet, I discovered that a change in hormones could cause this. Sure enough, after some time, when my testosterone levels stabilized, the palpitations lessened. And, as further proof, when my testosterone began to wane months later, I got a few palpitations again.

Later, I would also notice that my blood pressure fluctuated around when I got my pellets. During my peak testosterone levels, my BP was slightly higher, anywhere from five to ten points. When it was time for new pellets, when my testosterone levels dipped, my BP was down. When I graphed out my BP, I definitely saw a sine wave correlating to the dates of my pellet injections. Surprisingly, my cardiologist was not overly concerned, especially since I needed the pellets due to Low-T.

Eventually, I would change from pellets to testosterone gel. That kept my hormone levels more even-keeled, which also seemed to stop the heart palpitations.

Geez, I hated all of these issues.

CHAPTER 16: Fourth Year

My fourth year started out the same. My annual MRA went well, and the results showed nothing had changed. Which was great, because that meant I was still stable. Yes! Stable! What a wonderful, magical word for someone living with a critical condition. If you ever see someone react with joy to hearing the word "stable," they probably have gone through a major ordeal. Anyway, stable made me appreciate normalcy.

So, with things still going okay, Carole and I made plans for another overseas trip, this time to Israel. It was one of our bucket-list items. I was really getting more positive about things.

COVID-19

Then, 2020 hit.

Like most people, the start of the year was okay. Got through the holidays all right, and I just had my fifty-ninth birthday. But then there was all this talk about some virus way over in China. There wasn't much to worry about until the brunt of the coronavirus pandemic began. Then, as it was for everyone, a new way of life emerged. Just like with my health concerns, this was another instance of not realizing how good normalcy was until you no longer had it.

Luckily, my job allowed me to work from home, which was much more relaxing. That was good for my health. Plus, it gave me more time with Carole. And it allowed me to get an idea of what it would be like when I retired (which wasn't that far away). Being at home was also good for Carole, especially since I took over most of the cooking (something I really enjoy).

What wasn't so good was the stress and impacts brought on by the pandemic, which, for the most part, were the same type of issues faced by the vast majority of people. Like the fact that our bucket-list trip to Israel got canceled due to travel restrictions. (Luckily, we were able to defer it to the following year.) And even though being at home had its rewards, being isolated and scared to even go to the grocery store brought its own emotional toil. The panic and fear that was being generated about catching the virus was stupefying. I mean, who really goes around thinking that you might bring the virus into your home on the bottom of your shoes? Plus, who would have thought that the virus could cause heart and neurological problems? Personally, my worst fear of catching COVID-19 was the possibility of being put on a respirator in ICU, all alone, pretty much waiting to die.

COVID Vaccine

But considering how contagious COVID-19 was, it was mainly my health conditions that had me concerned. What was considered an underlying condition? Did having a dissection put me more at risk with the coronavirus? Initially, I was unsure if it was, because most information talked about lung and heart issues. Later, clearer information came out labeling aortic aneurysms and dissections as an underlying condition. It was lumped under coronary artery disease. But it didn't really matter anyway because my kidney disease definitely put me at risk. So, I decided it was best for me to get vaccinated. Afterward, I discovered that the mRNA vaccine caused some havoc to my kidneys. I'm still waiting to see if it is just temporary. Apparently, this was a "Damned if you do! Damned if you don't!" situation, at least for me. Either way, taking or not taking the vaccine appeared to be a gamble. I liked to think that I took the better odds.

Exercise and Yoga

Another impact from the pandemic was trying to keep up with exercising. With everything closed, I could no longer use our clubhouse exercise room. So, Carole and I adapted. First, we started walking two miles around our neighborhood every day, at a brisk pace. Second, we did what we could at home – twenty minutes of low weights or videos of yoga. However, I couldn't believe how out of shape I had become when trying to do simple yoga poses. I couldn't touch my toes anymore, and I could barely do poses requiring upper body strength. That was what you get when you become less active over the past four years. And here I thought I was doing fairly well.

Eventually, when the state of Texas began to reopen, Carole and I started doing yoga at our city's recreation center. But first, I wished to get approval from my cardiac surgeon, Dr. Reardon, to take senior yoga. I thought it would be okay, but I'd rather be safe. Dr. Reardon seemed amused that I was worried about senior yoga, but I don't think he understood that senior yoga can be a bit strenuous. Anyway, he told me that it was okay for me. In fact, he told me that based on my stability, I was well enough to do most physical things including sports, as long as I didn't overexert myself. I was surprised and elated to hear him say that. Good news.

Regardless, I tried to be very careful when I started out doing instructor-led yoga. I didn't want to overdo it. Which, at first, was a little embarrassing. But I couldn't let my pride risk my life. Hopefully, I would improve over time. Hopefully, I would at least be able to touch my toes again.

One thing that was part-good/part-bad was telemedicine. The good part was not having to take time to go to the doctor's office and spend more time waiting there. The bad part was that the doctor could not perform a physical examination, like listening to my heart or taking an EKG. For me I was doing fine enough that this wouldn't matter. That wasn't so fine for those people who really needed to be seen by a doctor.

Regardless, all of the back-and-forth news on the pandemic was quite confusing. If it weren't for the criticality of it, it'd be comical listening to the conflicting reports.

So, for the near future, life would be different. My hope was that this would resolve itself in 2021. Little did I know.

CHAPTER 17: Fifth Year

My fifth year went pretty much the same as my fourth year, which meant my MRA was still stable and there were no new issues (at least in regard to my dissection). The pandemic was still taking its toll, and I was still working from home. Since it didn't look like we would be able to travel anytime soon, at least internationally, we decided it was best to just give up on our trip to Israel, even though that meant losing quite a bit of money. The only good news was that some of my doctors started seeing their patients in person again. That made me feel better.

So, my aorta fears were lessening, and it was beginning to look like that my only significant health concern had to do with my kidneys (but that will have to be told in another book – thirty-plus years of kidney disease).

CHAPTER 18: Final Thoughts

Mokri Syndrome

An interesting side note:

One day, while reading someone's post on the Aorta Dissection Support Group on Facebook, there was a comment about a condition called Mokri Syndrome. I never heard of it before and none of my doctors ever mentioned it. I found out that it's a rare, progressive, supranuclear, palsy-like syndrome that occurs after thoracic aorta bypass surgery with deep hypothermia. That sounds familiar.

Symptoms include: a gaze palsy (like eyes not tracking), a gait imbalance (like constantly bumping into things), and dysarthria (motor speech disorder). Yep, sounds like me.

Some people with this syndrome also have epileptic seizures. That got me thinking. What if I have (had) this syndrome? Maybe this explains my near-fainting spells. Maybe my spells weren't from my ischemia. Hmmm. Looks like I should have had a conversation with my neurologist after all.

But, with my near-fainting spells seemingly gone, I'm not sure if I'll ever check into this. It could be that these seizures naturally faded away over time. This is all a bit scary. Only time will tell. If I start getting these spells again, then I'll schedule a trip to the doctor's office. Keeping my fingers crossed.

The Cost

I estimate that the cost of my event was well over one million dollars. And that doesn't include all the follow-ups (visits, tests, and procedures) and dealings with subsequent consequences (nosebleed surgery, TIA hospital stays, etc.). That could easily be hundreds of thousands of dollars more. The Methodist Hospital stay alone was around $600,000. Life Flight was around $25,000. Luckily, my out-of-pocket insurance maximum at the time was $2,000. If not for good insurance, Carole and I would be broke.

One thing odd was that I had to fight for Methodist Hospital to get paid by my insurance. For some reason, Methodist Hospital kept submitting their insurance claim incorrectly. Normally, I'd leave the hospital to fight for their money on their own, but their claim became a necessity for me on another claim. The rehab doctor for Methodist Hospital, Dr. Chan, was out-of-network. As such, my insurance paid him as out-of-network, which meant a few hundred dollars out of my pocket to cover the rest of his bill. Since neither Carole nor I requested Dr. Chan (he was directed by Methodist to see me), I contacted my insurance to explain the situation. In response, my insurance company agreed to pay Dr. Chan, but they said that they needed proof of my hospital stay at Methodist for the dates Dr. Chan billed me. Okaaay. I didn't understand why it wasn't evident that I was hospitalized, considering all the other medical bills already submitted, but my insurance company wouldn't budge until they received a finalized claim from Methodist Hospital that included hospital room charges for the dates in question. So, I went round and round between Methodist Hospital and my insurance company for months. In the meantime, I informed Dr. Chan's office of my situation and told them that I would not be paying them since they would eventually get money from my insurance. Well, years later, Methodist Hospital finally got their $600,000 bill resolved. Never heard back from Dr. Chan.

The Bad

So, at least for now, my biggest problem is emotional, not physical. For the first couple of years after my event, most days tended to be bad ones filled with anxiety, especially whenever I felt weird things in my chest (which used to be quite often, now I get them every now and them). Luckily, those days of bleakness have waned. Now, most days are good, *relatively*.

However, my near-death experience has caused me to become very self-conscious about life in general, and I'm reminded daily of my mortality, my frailty. I mean, we all know that we are going to die someday, but I think about it almost every day. It can become a bit depressing. I can't shake this worry, or this nagging thought, that somehow, I cheated death and it still lurks at my door. I yearn for the days of before when my thoughts were about the future, when I didn't look at my days as being numbered, and when I dreamt about all the things I hoped to do. Now, it's like having a shadow over me all the time. So, because of these dark thoughts, I often find myself wondering how many more years I really have left. But I am slowly learning to hand that concern over to God.

Also, like I've been saying throughout my story, this has definitely been a change in life not only for me, but also for Carole, who, by the way, is the only reason that I made it through this. I know that she has suffered in ways just as much as me. And, I have told her before that I'm not sure how I would have coped if the situation was reversed. It's scary enough to worry about your own life, but the thought of losing the one person you love the most is even scarier.

All in all, I am lucky to have survived such a high-percentage-morbidity event, and I am trudging forward to make the most of my second chance at life, or how I now look at it – my second life, because this new life is different than my previous life, not just in my restrictions, but also in my attitude.

And, I still have issues to deal with from my event. Some of these issues I expect will remain with me for the rest of my life.

On the emotional front, my PTSD has lessened, but I still find myself sensitive to emotional situations, and I still have some underlying resentment about my condition (which triggers an intolerant attitude and occasional temper tantrums). Even though I've become more aware of my outbursts, I still need to work on preventing them.

I still have trouble talking, especially when I get tired. The more tired my tongue gets, the more I slur my words. I also still have trouble coughing at night, which does not sit well with Carole since I constantly wake her up. The coughing is usually brought on by my gagging on saliva. That's because my weakened tongue still allows saliva to pass down my throat, even when just sitting around. The same problem affecting my tongue is also still causing me to continue biting the inside of my mouth, though the frequency of bites has declined.

My balance is still off. Besides being unable to run without falling, I have trouble dancing, and I keep running into things, especially our coffee table (damn malicious coffee table!). I have many leg bruises to show for it. Carole and I now laugh every time I bump into it. She'll say something like, "The coffee table is still there."

I also still have restrictions. *I will always have restrictions.* I can't ever do anything too strenuous or too physically aggressive, and I really need to be more aware of what stresses me out or gets me irritated. It's easy to become complacent when you feel good and have the strength. Again, my new normal.

The Good

But, all in all, my current impacts are very minor things to deal with considering what could have been, and not just that I could have died. I know that I am so lucky to have lived without any major complication, like being paralyzed from my stroke. That doesn't mean, though, that I still don't get depressed or angry over my situation. I think that it's natural to be upset when you have been dealt a major blow. Everything is relative. It's all in one's perspective.

And, speaking of perspective, one of the things that my event has taught me is to not take life for granted. Before, I kept thinking that I would have plenty of time to do the things I wanted to do. Now, I know there is no guarantee that I will have that time. In fact, due to my phobia of dying early, I don't feel that I have much time at all. The good in that is that I'm trying to focus on those things that are really important. This idea shouldn't be a revelation to anyone, but something has triggered in me to really embrace it.

I've also become a lot more spiritual (another greater positive coming from my event). Not religious, mind you, but spiritual in the sense that I've become closer to my image of God. I've always had my doubts about organized religions, being that they were created by men. So, I've come to build my relationship with God based on how I understand God, or at least what I think God should be like. This doesn't mean that I don't still have issues with faith. I'm just trying with all my might to trust God more, to trust God on pure faith. What helps is to put God into all the good that happens. I try to see God now in everything, from the major things like my surviving my event, to the smallest of things, like making it home safe from dinner out. As I keep hearing, if you are still alive, then God still has a purpose for you in this life. I wholeheartedly strive to believe that.

Finally, as with some others who experience trauma, my event seems to have brought Carole and me closer together. It's that cliché about not knowing what you really have until you almost lose it. It has strengthened our love, our bond. It's one of the greater positives I've experienced. For that, I am truly grateful, another gratitude given to God.

Looking Forward

With my aorta seemingly stable, I now need to be more focused on my other health issues. My aortic dissection is not the only critical item in my life. I also have Stage 4 chronic kidney disease (IGA Nephropathy), Barrett's esophagus (currently stable), and pre-cancerous colon polyps. It wouldn't do me much good to survive my dissection only to succumb to something else that I could have prevented. So, as I worry less about my aorta, my worry now tends to be more about my kidneys and the real future potential need for a transplant. Damn, life can be a pain.

~~~~~~~~~~~~~
~~~~~~~~~~~~~

So, in regard to my health, my goal is to survive long enough for my wife. With Carole being older than me, I don't need (or want) to live to a ripe old age (unless, of course, Carole lives for a very long time). No, I only wish to live to right past Carole's passing. So, if this aorta dissection shortens my lifespan, that's okay. As long as I can outlast Carole by one moment. I like to think that maybe God put this into my life to help me meet my goal.

My only other goal is to live a quality enough life that I will never become a burden to Carole. Having shortcomings is a part of life. What I'm talking about is that I hope that I never get to a physical or mental place that would cause undue hardship for Carole. I've already put her through enough with my health problems.

~~~~~~~~~~~~

So, after five years, I am filled with cautious hope. My last annual MRA was still good, which has prompted my cardiac surgeon, Dr. Reardon, to start having me come every two years for my MRA. My cardiologist was likewise happy with my last checkup and has told me that I only need to see him once a year, instead of every six months.

My stamina has returned, and I genuinely feel better. I'm still not sure how long my life expectancy is, but I figure that the longer I hold out, the better my chances are. I'm now to the point that I am actually beginning to make tentative plans for the long term. I'm even looking at writing more books, this time fictional stories. I can't keep wasting my time expecting the worst, expecting the other shoe to drop, so to speak. I don't know what God has in store for me, but that's the same for all people. My dire thoughts are still in the back of my mind, but for the most part, they don't control me anymore. At least it's progress.

So, my takeaway from all this is that an aortic dissection is survivable. And recovery is just a matter of acceptance and sometimes changing one's perspective. As the quote says, "We must be willing to let go
~~~~~~~~~~~~

of the life we planned, so as to accept the one that is waiting for us." For me, it is about maintaining focus on what's really important.

For those of you living with this condition or living with someone who has this condition, best wishes.

CHAPTER 19: What I've Learned

(Or, at least what I am trying to learn.)

- Sometimes, it's not until you lose even the most basic of things that you understand true gratitude for the things you have.
- Some things are neither good nor bad. It's just a matter of perspective.
- You are stronger than you think, when put to the test.
- From another aortic dissection survivor: "The ER doctor would rather see you twenty times and have it be nothing, than one time to see you dead."
- As one of my doctors told me: "I have to treat what will kill you first."

  When you have competing threats, deal with the one that is worst first. This is hard sometimes when dealing with multiple specialists who are more concerned with their particular area.

  As an example, I had to recently stop taking Lisinopril for my kidneys since it was causing my potassium to become dangerously high. Even though my kidneys may fail more quickly now, a high potassium can certainly kill me quicker.

- Having support makes the tough times easier. Lean on your family and friends.
- You (or your loved one) are your best patient advocate.

  It's not that the medical staff don't care, but they are human, and they make mistakes. Also, they don't always know what's best for you. You are not a medical statistic.

  Also, when you are unable to, your loved one can step in to ensure you have the best care. For me, Carole did an incredible job.

- Don't be afraid to ask questions. Lots of questions.
- Investigate who all might be part of any medical procedure as out-of-network staff/doctors are routinely brought in.

  This has happened to me several times and I wish it were illegal.

  As an example, when I went to the UTMB ER for my nosebleed, I checked in and was told that they accepted my insurance. Great! Later, I receive a bill from the ER doctor. Apparently, even though the hospital took my insurance, the ER doctor did not. He was out-of-network. Who would have rationally thought to ask if the hospital's ER doctor was on staff? Luckily, my insurance paid. This is absurd.

- The Internet is not absolute. Statistics are not absolute.

  Yes, we all know this, but when we are scared about our health condition and we don't get all the answers we want from our doctors, it is natural to look elsewhere.

  When I first looked into aortic dissections on the Internet, it scared the #$%@ out of me. All this talk about dying in a few years was very disturbing. The problem with the Internet is that you don't know where the data comes from or how it was collected. Much of the morbidity data on aortic dissections did not take into account what really killed the patient. Plus, the data was already outdated.

I really wish the medical staff spent more time with their patients going over all aspects of their condition.

- Medical staff also need to support a patient's emotional health.

  Our hospitals are great at emergency treatment, but they suffer when it comes to treating a patient's emotional trauma. PTSD, fear, depression, anxiety, and being overwhelmed by a critical event are real problems to be dealt with, but it's usually left to the patient to seek help.

  Don't be afraid to ask for help from someone, anyone.

4

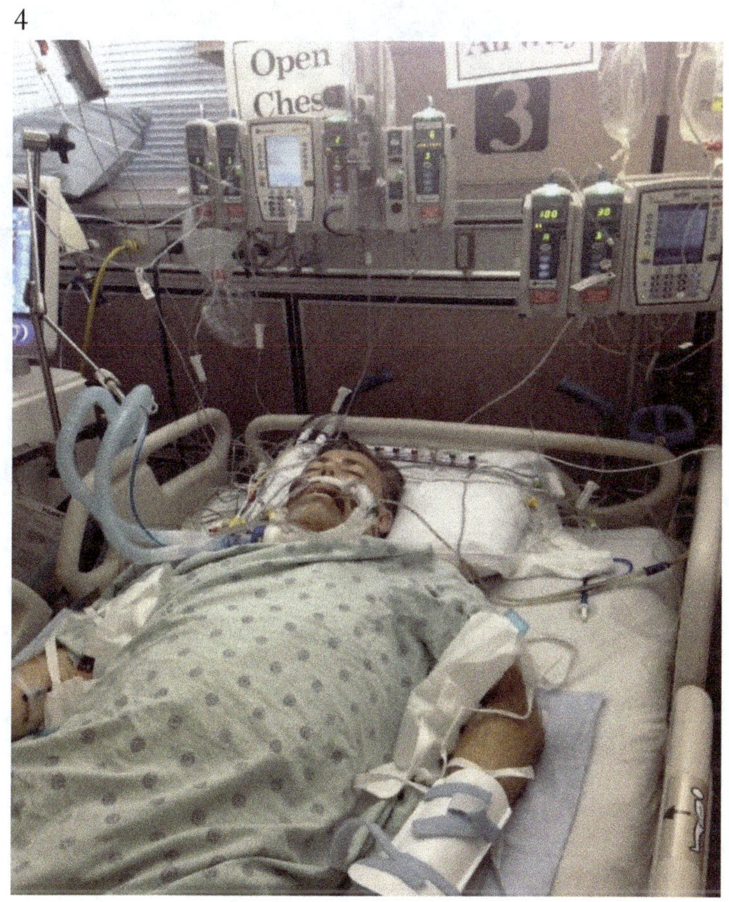

After surgery in critical care unit. Check out that "Open Chest" sign.

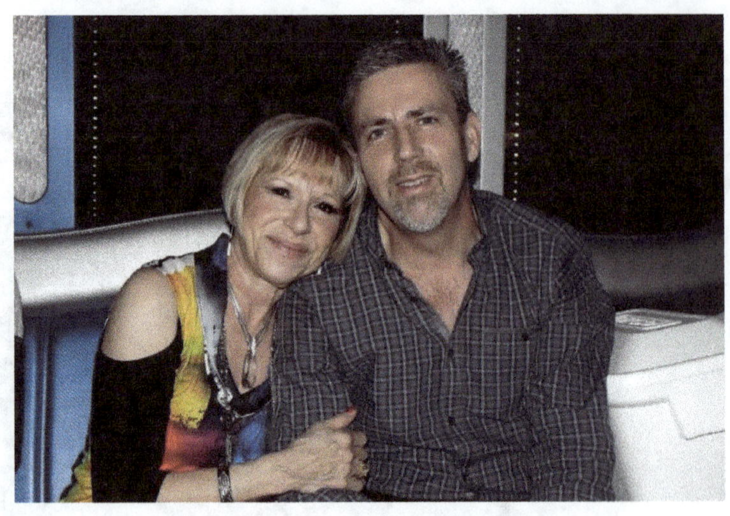

Me and my adorable wife, Carole, on a party bus with friends, celebrating her birthday and my recovery.

About the Author

Robert is the youngest of three children. Born in Sarnia, Ontario, Canada, he grew up with two older sisters, first in Chalmette, Louisiana, and later in Port Huron, Michigan. He graduated from Michigan Technological University in May of 1983. Traveling to the Houston, Texas area, he started his career as a software engineer in aerospace, working on the Space Shuttle and International Space Station projects. Today, he is retired with his wife, Carole, and his cat, Pippin.

Given a second chance, Robert no longer takes life for granted. With the premise that God is not done with him yet, his next goal is to continue with writing, this time fiction.

www.ingramcontent.com/pod-product-compliance
Lightning Source LLC
LaVergne TN
LVHW050415160826
845677LV00002BA/385